HIV
Test

The
HIV
Test

What You Need
to Know to Make
an Informed Decision

MARC VARGO, M.S.

POCKET BOOKS

New York   London   Toronto   Sydney   Tokyo   Singapore

The ideas, procedures, and suggestions in this book are intended to supplement, not replace, the medical advice of a trained healthcare professional. All matters regarding your health require medical supervision. Consult your physician before adopting the suggestions in this book, as well as any condition that may require diagnosis or medical attention. The author and publisher disclaim any liability arising directly or indirectly from the use of this book.

An *Original* publication of Pocket Books

POCKET BOOKS, a division of Simon & Schuster Inc.
1230 Avenue of the Americas, New York, NY 10020

Vargo, Marc.
    The HIV test : what you need to know to make an informed decision /
Marc Vargo.
        p.   cm.
    Includes bibliographical references.
    ISBN: 0-671-77950-8
    1.   HIV infections—Diagnosis.   2.   HIV infections—Diagnosis—
Psychological aspects. 3. AIDS (Disease)—Popular works. I. Title.
RC607.A26V36   1992
616.97'92075—dc20   92-14260
                                                                        CIP

First Pocket Books trade paperback printing September 1992

10   9   8   7   6   5   4   3   2   1

To Greg S. and the hundreds of HIV-positive men and women I have counseled in recent years through the NO/AIDS Task Force and the New Orleans AIDS Project. These people, having shared their innermost experiences with me, have taught me much about the extraordinary resilience, and the nobility, of the human spirit during times of trial.

Acknowledgments

I am deeply indebted to the following people, who were indispensable in the preparation of this book: Pamela Ahearn, of Southern Writers, for her encouragement and guidance from the inception of this project to its completion; Claire Zion, who served as executive editor for the book; Michael Sanders, the medical editor; Lisa Kazmier, assistant editor, who did a lot of the little jobs and was Fed Ex-er extraordinaire; Anne Cherry, the copy editor; and Diane Wilson, who provided assistance during critical periods of manuscript preparation.

I also wish to express my gratitude to Charles Cruce, whose patience and good humor sustained me during difficult periods of writing, and to Michael Vargo, for his support and encouragement throughout the project.

Marc Vargo
January 1992
New Orleans

Contents

Contents

Contents

Preface

by Roberta A. Bell, Ph.D.
*President, Neuropsychology Associates, Inc.,
New Orleans*

Have you been infected by the AIDS virus? To date, one out of every 135 Americans has been touched by this global epidemic, and most of them are unaware that they have contracted the virus. Unfortunately, all signs forewarn that the devastation wrought by this disorder will continue to escalate.

The HIV Test is the only sourcebook currently available that helps you assess your risk of infection by the human immunodeficiency virus (HIV) completely. Comprehensive and compassionately written, it provides the information you need to determine whether or not you should pursue testing. Should you indeed find that you have been infected, this guide offers further information and support to help you to begin to develop a healthy and adaptive perspective. Further, this compelling treatise assists you in adjusting to the news that a loved one or lover has become infected.

In the emergence of new drug treatments, which prolong both the duration and quality of life of people with HIV, the importance of early detection cannot be overemphasized. Before the century draws to a close, as many as forty million adults throughout the world may be struck by HIV infection. Thus, as conscientious people, we must avail ourselves of the most up-to-date and accurate information concerning the virus, its consequences, and its modes of detection and treatment.

Ultimately, the responsibility for your health is yours alone. To this end, the chapters that follow provide an unrivaled discussion and explanation of the state of the art of HIV testing.

The
HIV
Test

Introduction

In the mid-1970s, the United States was invaded by a lethal virus, an infectious agent that could attack and permanently destroy an individual's ability to combat any other illness or disease. By undermining the human immune system, this new, unidentified virus left its victims defenseless against almost any type of future infection or illness. Predictably, early studies suggested a very high mortality rate, as well as an alarming rise in the number of new cases being reported. Acquired Immune Deficiency Syndrome, or AIDS, was the term subsequently coined by the Centers for Disease Control in Atlanta to describe this formidable disease, and urgent public health warnings were issued in an effort to halt its spread.

Since that time significant advances have occurred in our understanding of AIDS. French and American teams, for instance, have now identified the Human Immunodeficiency Virus (HIV), and the medical community has developed laboratory tests that show if this virus is present in a person's body fluids or tissue—major breakthroughs in the diagnosis and treatment of HIV infection and its associated conditions, the first steps toward a cure. Known as HIV tests, these measures have proven to be remarkably accurate in detecting infection and are now in widespread use throughout the world.

Unfortunately, scientists up to now have been unable to create a vaccine capable of preventing infection with the virus. And while some experimental drugs show promise in slowing the course of the affliction, the cure is not yet in sight. The disheartening fact remains: HIV infection and AIDS, among the most menacing of modern-day illnesses, will most likely accompany us well into the next century. And it is for this reason that you, as an individual, must understand how to protect and preserve your own physical health and well-being during this ominous period.

First, you should thoroughly familiarize yourself with the manner in which the human immunodeficiency virus is transmitted. Since it is most often spread through specific behaviors, you need to understand these activities and avoid them. With a disease of this magnitude, there should be no compromises in your practice of a risk-free life-style.

Second, consider undergoing an HIV test to determine if you have already been infected with the virus. Such a test is extremely valuable if you have any suspicion that you might have been exposed, but you do have to be prepared to cope with test findings confirming this possibility. Indeed, coming to terms with positive test results can be an arduous task in itself, and the psychological element of the assessment process should not be underestimated.

In my experience as an HIV counselor, I always encourage people to express their feelings and thoughts when they first get their test results in order to gauge the direction and strength of their emotional reactions. As one would expect, their responses are frequently dramatic and intense.

Those who discover that they are not infected, for instance, react with elation and exuberance, while those whose findings suggest otherwise often respond with a sharp sense of catastrophe. Under such circumstances they interpret the test results as a symbolic death warrant and voice fears of mortality to the HIV counselor or physician. "It means I'm going to die," they will say. Of course, the findings do not automatically mean impending demise. But to the test recipient, the picture tends to look bleak, and a sense of doom often prevails. Emotional factors, then, assume a central role in an individual's manner of interpreting and adjusting to the test findings, and it is for this reason that a substantial portion of this book focuses on the psychological dimensions of HIV assessment.

In *The HIV Test,* you will learn the true nature of the infection: It is a long-term infection, which, in many cases, may be slowed or possibly arrested for an extended period of time with proper medication. I urge early HIV testing, so that treatment may be promptly initiated should the test findings indeed reveal the presence of infection.

Regarding the testing process itself, the book addresses the various tests currently in use, the types of facilities where an assessment may be performed, and the three types of findings that may emerge. Special attention is given to the emotional aftermath of a positive HIV test, including suggestions for coping with such information.

And finally, the effects of the test findings on others in one's life—family members or sexual partners—are discussed, with advice and guidance offered.

In essence, *The HIV Test* is designed to introduce you, the reader, to the assessment process and to sensitize you to its many ramifications—legal, emotional, social, and spiritual. In giving such a comprehensive presentation, I hope that your level of knowledge and personal awareness will be enhanced, thereby placing you in a sound position to plan realistically and responsibly for your future.

A wise man should consider that health
is the greatest of human blessings,
and learn how by his own thought
to derive benefit from his illnesses.

—Hippocrates
c. 460–400 B.C.

1

The Origin and Scope of the Global AIDS Epidemic

Since the dawn of time, the human race has struggled against the awesome and majestic forces of the natural world. Again and again we have attempted to conquer and harness the powers of nature in order to curtail their ability to inflict harm on us and to harvest their bountiful rewards. And yet, such a victory has been elusive. From widespread famine of centuries past to the great plagues that have ruthlessly stalked our people, the natural world has arbitrarily visited on us tides of destruction, demonstrating its ability both to create and to devastate. Such is the case with the Acquired Immune Deficiency Syndrome—AIDS—the most formidable disease to assail the human race in the twentieth century.

The first documented case of this fateful condition

occurred in England in the spring of 1959. A young British sailor developed an unusually violent illness that failed to respond to treatment by prominent medical specialists and resulted in his death within a year. Initially, he had developed skin lesions and gingivitis, but his symptoms soon multiplied, including fever, fatigue, shortness of breath, and weight loss. Medical tests also revealed the presence of two unusual infections, one a rare form of pneumonia previously found only in persons suffering from severely debilitating disease. No such underlying condition could be identified in the sailor, however (1). "We just didn't know what we were dealing with," Dr. George Williams, a physician associated with the case, later conceded (2).

So perplexed were doctors at the Royal Infirmary in Manchester that they sought the expertise of the President of the Royal College of Physicians, Sir Robert Platt, who recorded his concern in the patient's chart. Prophetically, this gentleman conveyed his fear that they might be witnessing the arrival of a new type of viral threat to the human species (3).

To focus still more attention on the disease, a detailed description was published in *Lancet,* a leading international medical journal. Providently, the doctors performed an autopsy, extracting and storing tissue samples in the hope of better understanding the enigmatic illness in the future.

In 1968, in St. Louis, Missouri, the tragic story was repeated: A fifteen-year-old boy is admitted to St. Louis City Hospital with extensive swelling of the lower extremities accompanied by fever. Though his medical treatment is prompt and aggressive, his condition spirals rapidly downward and he dies months later. An autopsy reveals the presence of a rare form of cancer, termed Kaposi's sarcoma, as well as several other medical anomalies. Puzzled by the unusual symptoms and relentless course of the syndrome, the youth's doctors freeze tissue and fluid samples, hoping that at some future time more sophisticated methods might help unravel the mysterious affliction (4).

Although similar cases have been reported in the medical literature, the two described here are of special merit, because of the specimens taken for later study. Recently, these samples were subjected to comprehensive clinical analysis, and the results proved to be enlightening.

In the autumn of 1989, research was begun on the tissue obtained from the sailor, using an innovative technique designed to detect the presence of the virus that produces AIDS. Eight months later, following extensive research in four independent laboratories, the findings revealed that the young Briton had, in fact, suffered from AIDS (5). Likewise, specialized blood tests confirmed that the St. Louis teenager had also been infected with the virus (6). In light of these findings, Dr. Williams, the British physician, concluded that HIV had "probably been stalking around the population for some time but lacked the momentum . . . necessary for it to create an epidemic." (7)

Indeed, other disturbing reports of a disease suggestive of AIDS date back to the beginning of the twentieth century, with exotic infections and obscure, devastating illnesses emerging unexpectedly and brutally in otherwise healthy European and American men. Applying the Centers for Disease Control's definition of AIDS, researchers have traced published reports of its apparent occurrence to 1902, when a cluster of seven cases was described in Italian men between that year and 1911. This grouping was followed by another twenty-two cases throughout Europe and the Americas between 1912 and 1966, with the victims being adult males in almost every instance (8). Additional episodes appear to have occurred in other parts of the world during the 1960s as well, most notably in equatorial Africa. And there is even evidence that the microbe was present in a remote Amazonian Indian tribe in Venezuela during this time (9). Finally, in the 1970s, an unprecedented AIDS epidemic erupted in Central Africa, which struck North America and Europe soon after.

Reviewing these events, it seems likely that this menacing virus has been with us, though hidden, for a long, long time. It has even been proposed that the microbe may be more ancient than the human race itself (10). The obvious question arises: Why, then, did HIV explode into an epidemic of worldwide dimensions at this particular moment in human history?

Of course, the precise reasons behind the abrupt and ubiquitous appearance of AIDS are unclear, but researchers believe that sweeping sociocultural changes in recent decades may have provided the precise conditions most conducive to its global spread. The ease and availability of international air travel, the invention and widespread use of hypodermic needles, the advent of blood transfusion techniques, and markedly increased sexual freedom—these have all been proposed as contributing to the proliferation of AIDS. Also noted is the uncanny relationship between the success of modern medicine in eliminating most other viral illnesses known to afflict the human species and the sudden appearance of this microbe. It has been suggested that by eradicating, or at least curtailing, these other "competing" infections, we may unwittingly have cleared the path for an even more powerful agent to invade and decimate our population (11). And finally, the virus may simply have evolved into a more violent, pernicious form through natural adaptive processes common to such organisms. Someday, through continued research, we will know why this happened.

We do know that the current North American epidemic began in the middle to late 1970s, with the first cases being publicly reported in June 1981. At that time the Centers of Disease Control (CDC), the epidemiological branch of the federal government, reported that five young homosexual men in the Los Angeles area had developed Pneumocystis pneumonia (12). One month later, the CDC issued another sobering report: Ten cases of Pneumocystis pneumonia, as well as twenty-six cases of Kaposi's sarcoma. Until that time, both illnesses had been extremely rare in the United States. As before, all involved homosexual men, with the latter report including men in New York as well as California (13). Thus, both coasts were hit; doctors and epidemiologists began to fear the outbreak of a new contagious disease.

Initially, due to their lack of familiarity with the condition, doctors were unable to understand or predict the course of the syndrome. "At first, I naively thought that the patients would recover and that they would be healthy once again," recalled Dr. Michael Gottlieb, one of the first physicians to discover and report the condition. "I was wrong. All of them died. It was clear to me before too long that we were on the brink of a natural disaster as devastating as any on earth" (14).

Also perplexing was the role played by sexual preference. Because young gay men were among the first casualties of this new affliction, some people believed that the syndrome was restricted to those of this sexual orientation. Accordingly, some observers came up with the misnomer Gay-Related Immune Deficiency, or GRID, to describe the condition. Unfortunately, this widely held but erroneous assumption would prove very damaging to both the heterosexual and homosexual populations. Many heterosexual men and women, assuming that they were not at risk, continued to engage in unsafe sexual activities and other risky behaviors, thereby exposing themselves to the virus. And the widely publicized link between this devastating disease and the gay life-style was used as ammunition by certain segments of the mainstream population in their fight against the homosexual presence: Gay men were now portrayed as pariahs. Futhermore, regardless of sexual preference, those suffering from AIDS frequently became the victims of intense cruelty, facing widespread rejection and discrimination in the community, the workplace, and even the medical setting itself. Thus, early in the North American epidemic, AIDS ceased to be viewed realistically as the appalling medical condition that it is and instead became, and remains today, a complex and divisive sociocultural phenomenon.

As the epidemic unfolded, it became increasingly evident that AIDS was *not* the exclusive province of homosexual men. Intravenous drug users were found to be infected in growing numbers, as were hemophiliacs—individuals with an inherited medical disorder necessitating frequent transfusions of blood or blood products. Furthermore, epidemiological research found certain racial minorities to have disproportionately elevated rates of AIDS, especially Hispanics and African-Americans,

Despite the obvious diversity among the individuals affected, however, society largely continued to treat those with the condition harshly.

Many individuals and organized groups persist in ostracizing and condemning those suffering from the disease, often blaming AIDS patients themselves for having contracted the grim illness and refusing to provide essential humanitarian support. In fact, the administration of President Ronald Reagan was widely accused of withholding desperately needed funds for medical research and public health education because the illness seemed to target only social, sexual, and racial minorities—groups not traditionally on the political A-list of the Republican Party. Indeed, many people now agree that the White House failed to provide sufficient monetary support until several years later, following profound and persistent criticism and political pressure from numerous sources, both within and outside the federal government. Meanwhile, tens of thousands of Americans contracted the lethal virus and growing numbers died.

The virus itself did not discriminate; as the epidemic flared across the nation, an even greater range of individuals was struck, among them heterosexual men, women, and their children. We learned, for example, that a pregnant woman infected with HIV could transmit the virus to the fetus during pregnancy or at the time of birth, thereby placing the child at significant risk for the later development of AIDS. In this manner, entire families could be destroyed. Thus, with the passage of time, we came to recognize the vast, aimless damage and waste the AIDS virus was inflicting on our people.

Still, paralleling the relentless march of the epidemic were impressive strides within the international research community. In 1983, Dr. Luc Montagnier and his colleagues at the Pasteur Institute in Paris discovered the virus that produces AIDS, now termed the Human Immunodeficiency Virus, or HIV (HIV-1). At the same time, and with the collaboration of the French researchers, an American team identified the same virus, with both groups eventually sharing joint credit for the momentous discovery.

Then, in 1985, a second breakthrough occurred with the advent of a laboratory test that indirectly measured the presence of the virus in the bloodstream—a crucial advance in the fight against AIDS. Because this test enabled us to determine whether an individual was infected, we have since become better able to protect our nation's blood supply from contaminated blood donations. Furthermore, because the test has proved reliable, economical, and versatile, it has been used extensively in a number of other settings as well. In cities throughout the country, assessment programs are now in place that allow an individual to be tested under voluntary, anonymous conditions—an essential step when planning a pregnancy or determining the need for medical treatment for HIV infection. Thus, while a cure has not been forthcoming, at least a feasible means of determining the existence of infection *is* available, and the test is being used routinely throughout the world.

In addition, progress in the medical sphere has produced drugs capable of slowing or temporarily arresting the virus's reproduction in an individual's body, delaying the onset of symptoms for months or years. Innovative treatments enhancing the longevity and quality of life of HIV-infected persons have also been created to address many of the opportunistic infections that so often afflict them. In all, then, the outlook for those infected with the virus has steadily improved since HIV first burst forth a decade ago, and there is every reason to believe that such advancements will continue and even accelerate in the years ahead.

Regarding society itself, while the epidemic initially brought widespread stigmatization and bias, in recent times the crisis has given rise, in some quarters, to wisdom, maturity, and benevolence. From Washington, D.C., to the Vatican, many national and international bodies have protested the insensitivity to which AIDS patients have been subjected and have called for their equitable, judicious, and humane treatment. Such insistent pleas have often been surprisingly effective in ensuring the rights of those affected by the epidemic.

To date, nearly 180,000 Americans have been diagnosed as having symptoms of AIDS (15), while up to one million are believed to be harboring the virus in their bodies, often without symptoms (16). Trends indicate that AIDS will soon be the second leading cause of death of American men between the ages of twenty-five and forty-four, and may become one of the five primary causes of death of women between the ages of fifteen and forty-four (17). The Centers for Disease Control further predict that 40,000 new HIV infections will occur each coming year in adolescents and adults, along with 2,000 infections in newborns (18).

On the global stage, over 370,000 AIDS cases have been reported in 163 nations (19). The World Health Organization predicts that during the 1990s, the total number of adult cases of HIV infection will reach an astounding forty million, with several hundred thousand of these infections progressing to AIDS before the turn of the century (20). Clearly, this extraordinary epidemic will have a profound impact on the next generation: Ten million children are predicted to lose one or both parents to AIDS by the end of this decade (21).

The limited progress we are making against the epidemic can be seen in recent, significant changes in the populations it targets. Whereas in the United States, the disease initially appeared to have an affinity for gay men and blood transfusion recipients, the number of new infections within these groups is decreasing; instead, the infection rate is now rising among children and adolescents, racial minorities, and the poor and disenfranchised. In Western Europe, the total number of AIDS cases continues to climb, and it is feared that the recent political liberation of Eastern Europe may lead to increased vulnerability in these nations as well. In equatorial Africa, the epidemic rages unabated. And worsening the situation further still is the emergence in western parts of that continent of a second strain of the virus, HIV-2, which is equally destructive in its effects and which is currently exacting a staggering toll.

It is therefore essential that we understand and respect the leviathan dimensions of this international health threat and the utter devastation it may wreak in the lives of millions. Unfortunately, because of the myriad factors that influence viral spread, it is exceedingly difficult to predict the precise path this worldwide epidemic will take, just as it is beyond our ability to foresee with certainty its medical, legal, and sociocultural consequences. Instead, we can only trust that the spread of the virus will ebb at some point, due either to natural processes or to our own scientific achievements.

Until that time, it is up to you, as a responsible individual, to protect yourself and others from contracting the virus. You must understand the ways in which it is transmitted and rigorously avoid those activities deemed potentially dangerous. And if you have reason to suspect that you have already been in contact with HIV, you should consider undergoing a blood test to determine whether you are infected, since it is only through an actual laboratory analysis that the condition can be confirmed. If you are infected, you should seek ambitious medical treatment to control the condition as much as possible.

In this age of AIDS, testing and follow-up medical treatment are both readily available in most communities, and you would be well advised to avail yourself of such potentially life-extending measures. To this end, this book is designed to inform and assist you during this important process, to serve as your guide through the labyrinth of issues and concerns that come with medical testing for HIV infection.

2

Risk Factors for
HIV Infection

During the past ten years we have learned an enormous amount about the human immunodeficiency virus and the means by which it is spread. Contrary to popular belief, we have found that it is not an easy virus to contract.

We know that HIV is a blood-borne microbe that exists in specific body fluids and is spread chiefly through penetrative sexual acts like anal and vaginal intercourse, intravenous drug use, and from mother to child during pregnancy and especially during delivery. We know, too, that most such behaviors are voluntary, and that a person may choose to participate in them or may modify or discontinue them. Thus, infection is largely preventable. In addition, because research has yielded a comprehensive index of infectious activities, anyone can now determine the possi-

18

bility of his or her prior contact with the virus by recalling and evaluating risk-related behaviors they may have engaged in since the middle to late 1970s, the period when the American epidemic is believed to have begun. As a result, you should be able to make a relatively well-informed decision about whether or not you need HIV testing.

To help you, here we will review the means by which the virus is transmitted. Specifically, we will discuss potentially infectious sexual and reproductive activities, including heterosexual and homosexual practices, artificial insemination, pregnancy, and childbirth; medical procedures, such as blood transfusions, organ transplants, and "traditional" medical practices from other cultures; accidents in the medical workplace; and intravenous drug use. We will also review other factors believed to contribute in some manner to the contraction of the infection. The chapter concludes with a discussion of the means by which HIV is *not* spread, to dispel any unfounded anxieties or concerns you may have.

Before we begin, however, it is important for you to understand that simply having engaged in a "risky" behavior does not, in itself, signify that you are infected with the virus. Indeed, some individuals have repeatedly participated in an array of unsafe activities with HIV-infected partners, yet apparently have not contracted the infection. Of course, others have acquired it after only a single incident. It is for this reason that you must undergo an HIV test if you wish to know with certainty whether you are infected. But first, you must determine if you have participated in any of those potentially hazardous practices that would indicate the need for such a test.

Sexual Acts

The human immunodeficiency virus can be found in numerous body substances like saliva, tears, and urine, but in very low quantities—so low, in fact, as possibly to be harmless. The virus does exist in much higher, infectious amounts in three other types of fluids, however: in high concentrations in blood, and to substantial degrees in semen and vaginal secretions. Since these particular substances may be present in significant amounts during sexual activity, physical intimacy may be especially hazardous if either partner is infected.

Statistics from the Centers for Disease Control reveal 65 percent of Americans infected with HIV contracted it through sexual activity (1). It is ironic, then, that one of the most alluring and joyful experiences in human life—sexual union—may now be dangerous under certain conditions. And specific sexual practices may be harmful regardless of whether they occur between members of the same sex or the opposite sex, since it is the nature of the act itself rather than the gender of the participants that creates the conditions for infection. For the sake of clarity, however, we will discuss the activities of the principal sexual orientations separately.

SEXUAL RELATIONS BETWEEN MEN

When men engage in sexual relations together, some choose the act of anal intercourse. Though gratifying, this particular act may be extremely perilous since it is, of all forms of sexual expression, the one that carries the highest threat of infection, especially for the passive (receptive) partner. Since the lining of the anal passage may easily be torn or sustain other abrasions that bleed during intercourse, there is a direct route of viral entry into the bloodstream of the passive partner through the mucous membrane. It should be noted, too, that the active partner is also at risk, because the virus may enter his penis through the urethra to produce infection.

If you have engaged in anal intercourse in recent years as either an active or passive partner, it is possible that you may have come into contact with the virus. This is especially true if you were with a person known to be infected with HIV or one whose HIV status was unknown to you. Also, your chances are heightened if you have engaged in this practice frequently or with multiple partners. And finally, the threat is obviously much greater if no condom or anti-HIV lubricant (e.g., nonoxynol-9, a substance that kills the virus) was used during intercourse, or if a condom ruptured or leaked during the sex act. When determining your need for HIV testing, then, these factors should also be taken into consideration.

Concerning another common form of sexual expression—oral intercourse—we still cannot say with certainty the degree of risk involved, since it has yet to be reliably determined. During oral sex, the person performing the act may receive his partner's preseminal fluid in the mouth; a substance that could possibly be infectious. The individual may also receive the partner's semen in his mouth, and semen is definitely infectious. Thus, if the man performing the act were to have cuts or abrasions in his mouth, theoretically the partner's body fluids could enter the man's bloodstream through such portals and infect him. Possibly, the lining of the mouth itself could absorb the infectious fluids, even in the absence of such abrasions. The chances of contracting the virus through oral sex are increased if the person conducting the act regularly receives his partner's ejaculate in his mouth, if the act is performed frequently, and if there are a number of different partners to whom one is exposed.

As for the passive partner in oral sex, again, we do not know for certain whether a significant risk is present, but we should assume that at least the possibility exists. Although the amount of virus in human saliva is extremely low, and while there are studies indicating that certain chemicals in saliva may actually render the virus inactive (2), we cannot categorically rule out oral sex as a route of viral transmission.

It should be recognized, too, that the person performing the act may have small amounts of blood in his mouth due to many reasons (e.g., gum disease), and that this blood may come into direct contact with the penis of the receptive partner. Clearly, this places the receptive partner at risk.

To reiterate, it has not been firmly established that HIV infection can be contracted by receptive oral sex; more research is needed before we can determine the actual degree of risk involved in this practice.

And finally, among those forms of same-sex activities generally considered to be free of significant risk is mutual masturbation, a practice whereby the partners manually stimulate each other to orgasm. During this act, the threat of infection is negligible, since semen does not enter the body of either man. As long as infectious fluids remain outside the body, they are harmless, since unbroken skin is considered to serve as an effective barrier against the human immunodeficiency virus.

SEXUAL RELATIONS BETWEEN WOMEN

When women make love to one another, a common form of sexual expression is oral sex and, as in heterosexual couplings, some degree of risk may be present, especially if performed during menstruation.

Since women having sex together do not engage in actual vaginal or anal intercourse, lesbian practices carry less risk of HIV transmission than some of the more common male homosexual or heterosexual practices—a fact that has been evident since the early years of the epidemic. Still, a threat may exist, especially if the women share sexual toys or devices to simulate intercourse, since these objects may constitute a source of viral transmission. Of course, the same threat is posed between two men or within a heterosexual coupling when toys or devices containing partners' body fluids are shared.

SEXUAL RELATIONS BETWEEN MEN AND WOMEN

A sense of intimate union between a man and woman is typically achieved through sexual intercourse—most frequently vaginal intercourse, although a certain portion of couples engage in anal sex as well, at least occasionally.

During vaginal intercourse, there is a somewhat greater chance that the woman will become infected rather than the man. This may reflect the much larger pool of men in our population who are currently infected with HIV, thereby placing the woman at increased odds of encountering an infected sexual partner. Yet it is essential to remember that both the male and female are at potential risk of HIV infection during this sexual practice.

To evaluate your need for HIV testing based on vaginal or anal intercourse, you should consider whether you have reason to believe that your partner may have been infected at the time you engaged in sex together. Also pertinent is the number of occasions on which you have had intercourse with a potentially infected partner, the overall number of different partners you have had in recent years, and the consistency with which you have used condoms or an anti-HIV spermicide (e.g., nonoxynol-9) when being intimate. For a man, an additional risk is involved in having intercourse with a woman during her menstrual period, thus exposing him to blood.

In oral sex, a woman performing oral intercourse on a man may be at risk for infection if she receives the man's preseminal fluid or semen in her mouth, since these secretions may enter the mucous membranes lining the inside of her mouth and make their way into her bloodstream. A man performing oral sex on a woman may be at risk also, since he will come into contact with vaginal fluids that may contain the virus. Of course, if he performs this act during the woman's menstrual period, his chances of contracting the virus may be enhanced.

As with oral sex between two men or two women, heterosexual oral sex may or may not present a significant hazard; the actual degree of risk has yet to be determined. Nevertheless, due to the profound consequences if oral sex does prove to be an infectious practice, one would be well advised to take sufficient precautions when engaging in this activity.

In terms of the need for HIV testing, male–female oral sex is considered to carry a potential risk of infection. Generally, though, it is not believed to be as great as that associated with unprotected vaginal or anal intercourse.

Masturbation between a man and a woman is usually

considered to be a harmless activity, since one's semen, blood, or vaginal secretions do not typically enter the partner's body. Intact skin normally serves as an effective barrier against HIV infection.

Although heterosexual contact accounts for only 4 percent of the total number of AIDS cases in the United States, this percentage represents thousands of infected persons. Futhermore, the number of cases contracted through heterosexual practices has tripled in the past decade, despite extensive public education campaigns designed to promote safer sex. Judging from such patterns, male–female transmission is expected to rise in the coming years, thus increasing any individual's chances of meeting an infected partner. Such disturbing trends underscore the need for sensibility and caution during sexual encounters.

ASSOCIATED SEXUAL PRACTICES

Across all sexual orientations, a common form of physical intimacy involves deep kissing, also referred to as "French" or "wet" kissing. Like any other sexual activity that involves the intake of a partner's body fluids, this form of sexual expression cannot be ruled out as a form of viral transmission, even though there has never been a documented case in which a person contracted HIV in this manner. Because saliva may be exchanged in substantial amounts during deep kissing, if this substance were eventually determined to be infectious under certain conditions, then HIV could conceivably be spread in this way. The question is, of course, whether saliva is infectious, and under what circumstances. At present, it continues to be a source of debate within the scientific community.

In recent years, researchers have detected the presence of antibody to HIV in the saliva of infected individuals, but no study has been able to detect actively infectious virus itself in this fluid. Research conducted by Siobhan O'Shea and associates, for example, measured the amount of infectious virus in several body fluids obtained from HIV-positive individuals, and found it in the blood, semen, and vaginal fluids of many of the participants (3). Infectious virus was not found in the participants' saliva, however. These researchers concluded that either HIV is neutralized by enzymes present in saliva and is therefore unable to survive in this fluid or the amount of infectious virus is so low as to be unmeasurable by their methods. Thus, the available evidence suggests that saliva is much less infectious than other bodily substances, a conclusion supported by the zero incidence of transmission through casual contact in the home and hospital.

Other low-risk or risk-free activities include dry or "social" kissing, which involves a very limited exchange of saliva. Also harmless are those practices restricted to external skin contact if the skin is healthy and unbroken. Such activities include hugging, caressing, and "frottage," or body-to-body rubbing.

Finally, there are those exotic sexual practices that may possess varying degrees of risk. Some forms of sadomasochism, such as bondage and flagellation, may be potentially infectious, since they may involve the presence of blood. Similarly, the practice of "rimming"—the oral stimulation of a partner's anal region—may be risky, because it may entail contact with substances containing the virus. Essentially, any sexual activity in which the blood, semen, or vaginal fluids of one person enter into the body of another is potentially infectious and may, depending upon the circumstances, justify HIV testing.

Perinatal Transmission

Because the human immunodeficiency virus is transported by semen, blood, and related substances, it may be spread through natural or artificial insemination, thereby producing infection in a woman. During the resultant pregnancy, she may unknowingly transmit the virus to her child in utero or especially during birth. A woman considering pregnancy should therefore clearly understand the risks involved in HIV infection before proceeding, and is further advised to seek HIV testing before embarking on such a consequential event.

ARTIFICIAL INSEMINATION

The medical procedure of artificial insemination involves the nonsexual introduction of a male donor's sperm into a woman's body. This technique has found widespread acceptance in the treatment of infertility and has become a relatively common practice in the United States and other nations. Unfortunately, artificial insemination has also been found to lead to HIV infection in some cases.

In a study of 134 women who inadvertently received sperm donations from HIV-infected men, subsequent antibody testing revealed that one of the women had become infected with the virus (4). Another study found a much higher rate of infection, possibly because the women in this investigation had received a larger number of sperm samples (5).

To resolve the problem of infected donations, it is very likely that, in the future, domestic clinics that practice insemination techniques will increasingly comply with the Centers for Disease Control's recommendations for the routine antibody screening of all potential donors, as well as the use of associated protective methods. If you are a woman having concerns about the insemination procedure, you might wish to contact the facility at which you underwent, or plan to undergo, artificial insemination, to evaluate its policies and practices regarding the HIV-antibody testing of its donors, as well as any other procedures it may employ to safeguard the health of its clientele.

PREGNANCY AND CHILDBIRTH

An HIV-infected pregnant woman stands a significant chance of passing the infection to her infant, a form of viral transmission that accounts for 1 percent of American AIDS cases (6). During pregnancy, it appears that the fetus may become infected through placental transfer or during the birth process itself, when exposure to the mother's mucus and blood is greatest.

Researchers at the National Cancer Institute, reviewing medical data collected on sixty-six sets of twins, found that the firstborn twin—the one having the heaviest contact with the mother's fluids during delivery—was more than twice as likely to be infected with HIV than the second-born twin. Even when delivery was by Caesarian section, firstborns were infected much more often, a finding strongly suggesting that childbirth is an important source of HIV infection.

To address this problem, the researchers recommended that further studies be conducted to determine whether cleansing the birth canal with anti-HIV agents prior to vaginal delivery would decrease the chances of viral transmission. Also, they want to investigate whether a Caesarian section performed before membrane rupture would decrease the possibility of infection (7).

Other studies have tracked the antibody status of HIV-positive infants during the first months and years of life. Interestingly, many newborns who initially possess an antibody to HIV eventually shed it from their systems and then test negative. This suggests that the infants were not actually infected; the antibody detected by the tests was a "maternal" antibody passed on during pregnancy.

In this regard, a large-scale investigation, the European Collaborative Study, examined 600 newborns of HIV-infected mothers and found that 343 of these neonates initially tested positive on antibody tests. Eighteen months later, only 64 continued to test positive (13 percent). Hence, the majority discarded their antibody to HIV, suggesting that they were never truly infected (8).

Finally, it has been reported that healthy, uninfected infants of HIV-positive mothers may possibly be at a mild risk of later contracting the virus, if they ingest the mother's infected breast milk (9). However, further research is needed before we can state with certainty and precision the actual degree of risk involved in this practice.

If you are planning a pregnancy and have reason to believe that you may have been in contact with the virus, you are advised to seek HIV testing before proceeding. If you do indeed carry the virus, it is very strongly recommended that you postpone the pregnancy until more is understood about *in utero* HIV infection.

If you're already pregnant and find out you're infected, you should consult your physician or others whose judgment you respect and examine the options available to you. Because the health risks involved are so serious, alternatives such as timely pregnancy termination may well be valid considerations. And if you decide to continue the pregnancy, close medical supervision throughout its course and afterward is essential to keep you and your child healthy.

In all, if you are pregnant and HIV-infected, you will face many complex issues for which there is often no easy resolution. Since the powerful concept of motherhood is involved, both familial and sociocultural expectations and pressures may impinge on you, sharply etching your choices and complicating your decisions. If you should find yourself in such a disheartening situation, consider seeking support and assistance from a mental health center, medical agency, community AIDS center, or a women's support organization. During such potentially confusing and turbulent times, concerned and effective guidance can be extremely beneficial in helping you plan soundly for your future.

Transfusions, Transplants, and Traditional Medicine

A few years ago, it became apparent that HIV infection could be contracted through the receipt of a contaminated blood transfusion, a source of infection to which our population was especially vulnerable during the early years of the epidemic. At one point, approximately 4 percent of all AIDS cases in the United States were the result of contaminated blood transfusions or other tainted blood products (10). Today, all potential donors are tested for HIV infection, and certain concentrated blood products are even heat treated to insure their purity. As a result, our national blood supply is now much more secure.

If you received a blood transfusion between the mid-1970s and the mid-1980s, however, and particularly if you lived in an urban area with pronounced rates of early AIDS cases (New York City, Los Angeles, San Francisco), you might consider discussing the need for an antibody test with an HIV counselor or physician. While the chances are low that you are infected, it is still a possibility that you might wish to explore.

At this juncture, it should be emphasized that an individual cannot acquire HIV infection by *donating* blood. Apparently there is confusion among the public regarding the act of giving blood and the contraction of HIV infection. The facts are very simple: Disposable needles are used to draw blood in the United States and are discarded after a single use; therefore, absolutely no risk exists for the donor.

In terms of tissue transplant procedures, several cases of HIV infection resulting from this practice have been documented. The transplantation of internal organs, including kidney, heart, and liver, as well as bone, have been reported as the cause of infection in the recipient (11). Fortunately, with the advent of routine antibody testing of organ donors in the mid-1980s, such risks have been sharply reduced. If, however, you underwent an organ or bone transplant between the mid-1970s and the mid-1980s, then you might discuss the situation with your physician to determine if HIV testing is advisable.

Finally, in other cultures, traditional medical procedures exist that may contribute to HIV infection. For instance, a case has been reported in which infection was spread through the Chinese practice of acupuncture (12). In more primitive societies, traditional medical practices such as ritual circumcision and the various forms of ceremonial tattooing, scarring, and skin piercing have also been proposed as promoting the spread of the virus (13).

Risks in the Health Care Setting

There are certain professions that, by their nature, put a person in close proximity to the human immunodeficiency virus. Health care workers—nurses, physicians, dentists, emergency medical technicians, and laboratory technicians—comprise a group that is especially vulnerable to viral exposure.

A small number of cases has been reported in which health care workers have been infected with HIV in the workplace, either from needlestick injuries or through exposure of the mucous membranes or impaired skin to large amounts of patients' infected blood. By and large, however, most such cases could have been prevented had the workers followed standard precautions for infection control.

Currently, the chances of contracting the virus through needlestick injury or exposure of mucous membranes to infected fluids are less than one-half of 1 percent (14)—reassuring figures to those in the health care professions. Still, the possibility of infection does exist, and you should be cautious if you work in this environment. The Centers for Disease Control have issued guidelines for medical personnel to follow in the event of certain types of work-related accidents involving HIV-infected patients. Under certain circumstances, the recommendations include the antibody testing of the worker (15). If you are a health care professional and believe that you may have been exposed on the job, you should obtain these guidelines from your organization and follow their recommendations.

The Sharing of Hypodermic Needles

Within certain populations, the primary means by which the human immunodeficiency virus is transmitted is through sharing hypodermic needles during drug use. Indeed, the virus can easily be injected directly into one's bloodstream through the use of a contaminated needle, whether the route of entry is intravenous, intramuscular, or subcutaneous.

Sharing contaminated needles accounts for 27 percent of all AIDS cases in the United States (16), a figure currently on the rise. Furthermore, this means of transmission is most prevalent within the Hispanic and African-American communities—a fact that concerns health educators because these groups are among the most difficult to reach. In some respects, the values and customs of minority communities are different from those of the mainstream population. As a result, public health campaigns designed for the general population are not always effective. It appears, too, that drug users may pass the virus to their sexual partners and, eventually, through pregnancy and childbirth, to their children. Entire families may thus become infected.

If you inject drugs, you may be at risk for HIV infection if, in recent years, you have injected yourself with a hypodermic needle used by another individual but not disinfected between uses. Unless you know with absolute certainty that the person with whom you shared was not HIV-infected, then you should consider seeking a test. Of course, under the influence of the drug, you may not remember with whom, or even if, you shared a needle. Obviously, you should still consider being tested.

Similarly, if you are, or may have been, the sexual partner of an IV drug user, testing should be a consideration if you had unprotected sex—if the person's blood, semen, or vaginal fluids came into direct contact with impaired skin on your body (e.g., cut, burned, or chapped skin). For example, vaginal or anal intercourse with an intravenous drug user, because of the person's possible history of needle sharing, clearly increases your own chances of HIV infection.

Contributing Factors in HIV Infection

In addition to behaviors that may produce HIV infection, there are other factors also associated with viral transmission. For instance, a relationship has been found between HIV infection and a personal history of other sexually transmitted diseases (17). Also, the infectious state of the carrier—the person who infects another—may be critical in HIV transmission. It has been proposed that, as the carrier's HIV infection progresses, a gradual increase may occur in the actual amount of virus in the person's system, rendering the individual increasingly more infectious with the passage of time. It has been hypothesized, too, that some strains of HIV may be more virulent than others. And research findings suggest that a certain genetic predisposition may exist that affects one's susceptibility to HIV infection [18, 19]. Finally, the preexisting state of health of the person exposed to the virus may be critical; if one's immune system is already impaired due to other types of infection or illness, the person may be more vulnerable to the effects of HIV than the individual whose immune system is intact and functioning optimally.

Ways in Which the Virus Is Not Transmitted

Because so many in our society have overreacted during this disturbing epidemic, it cannot be emphasized enough that basic social contact with those infected with HIV or having symptoms of AIDS is harmless. We now have a decade of clinical and epidemiological research to draw upon, and it clearly shows the key ways in which this virus is and is not spread. Virtually all common social practices have been found to be very safe indeed.

The virus, although extraordinarily potent while in a person's bloodstream, is quite fragile when it is no longer in the human body. Once it is in the external environment, HIV can be killed quickly and easily with hydrogen peroxide or a bleach solution.

In terms of contagion, HIV is actually fairly hard to contract. You cannot contract HIV from activities involving only skin-to-skin contact, such as shaking hands, embracing, hugging, massage, or contact sports. You cannot contract it by breathing the air in a room shared with an infected person, working in the same office, sharing office equipment, or attending public events together. You cannot contract the virus from food prepared by a chef who is infected, or by eating from the plate or drinking from the glass of an infected person. Indeed, the *Surgeon General's Report on Acquired Immune Deficiency Syndrome* concludes that eating utensils, including straws and dishes, can be shared without risk of infection (20). Still, common sense dictates that one should not share razors, toothbrushes, or other such objects, since these may contain minute quantities of blood that could conceivably infect the user.

You cannot contract HIV by swimming in a pool with an infected person or by sharing a hot tub, whirlpool, or sauna. Household furniture, rest room facilities, and doorknobs also carry no risk of infection. And, while certain types of insects (i.e., mosquitoes) do transmit specific diseases to humans, at no point in this epidemic has a case of HIV infection been found to occur in this manner. Consequently, insects are not believed to constitute a risk, nor are domestic pets, such as dogs, cats, or other animals.

Because so many factors, some still a mystery to us, may contribute to the contraction of the virus, the only way to determine with certainty whether you have HIV is to be tested. If you have engaged in the past few years in practices known or suspected to be risky, you are advised to consider undergoing an assessment. In addition to the issues discussed in this chapter, you should also understand the nature of HIV testing itself and give serious thought to relevant medical, legal, and emotional aspects when planning your assessment. These issues are discussed in following chapters.

3

The Practice of HIV Testing

Today we have at our disposal an array of tests for HIV. Some of these detect the presence of the virus in the body; others gauge the body's reaction to it. In this chapter, both types will be described, followed by a review of the various clinical settings in which an individual may undergo such tests. We will also discuss when to seek an assessment, with emphasis placed on the advantages of early testing. We begin by briefly reviewing the nature and functioning of the human immune system, essential knowledge for understanding the HIV testing process.

The Immune System

An impressive structure, the human immune system protects an individual's health and well-being by fighting diseases that threaten the body. When an aggressive agent, such as a virus, enters a person's bloodstream, it is the immune system that detects the presence of the intruder and mounts an attack against it. Normally, this is rapidly accomplished through the creation of anti-body—agents produced by the body to eliminate intruding germs. For each type of intruder, the immune system creates a highly specific antibody to kill it. Once they have successfully completed their mission, the antibodies may remain in the bloodstream.

Unfortunately, when HIV infiltrates the system, a unique and apparently irreversible process occurs. First, the virus typically exists for several weeks or months in the bloodstream before the body even detects it and begins forming antibody to fight it. Thus, a lengthy delay occurs before the immune system responds to the threat. Second, the virus specifically attacks critical cells within the immune system—the very cells that would normally mount a defense against it. And finally, for reasons not yet understood, the specific antibody appears unable to destroy the human immunodeficiency virus. Consequently, it is believed that, once infected, a person remains infected for life.

SYMPTOMS OF INFECTION

When the virus initially enters the bloodstream, no noticeable symptoms occur. Weeks or months later, however, as the body detects the virus and activates a defense against it, some individuals experience a short-lived illness. The symptoms often include skin rash, sore throat, muscular aches, swollen lymph nodes, diarrhea, fever, fatigue, and malaise. Typically self-limiting, this fleeting illness usually abates within a few days. It is important to note, however, that these symptoms, referred to collectively as "acute infection illness," do not comprise AIDS, nor are they exclusive to HIV infection; they may be present in many other infections as well, such as influenza or mononucleosis.

Once the symptoms subside, if they occur at all, an extended symptom-free period usually ensues, during which the virus lives, silently, for several years within the body. Although not yet proven, it is conceivable that some persons infected with HIV may live in fine health with the virus in their bodies for the rest of their lives. Unfortunately, many do not, instead developing chronic symptoms at some point, primarily in the form of an inability to resist effectively various illnesses and infections. If it progresses, such an erosion of immunological functioning may eventually culminate in Acquired Immune Deficiency Syndrome.

Although we generally refer to AIDS as a disease or an illness, in actuality it is neither. It is a *condition* or *state* of profound defenselessness, which renders an individual vulnerable to disease or illness. And since the immune system is damaged, any number of maladies may threaten it, especially infections resulting from invasion by hostile microbes. Such illnesses, termed "opportunistic infections," are particularly troublesome for persons with AIDS and account for some of their most persistent medical problems. Furthermore, repeated infections in a person having AIDS may overwhelm and ultimately exhaust the immune system, making recovery difficult.

Types of HIV Tests

The human immunodeficiency virus is an incredibly small organism, so small that most laboratories are not equipped to measure directly its presence in a blood sample. Instead, they test for the existence of the antibody the immune system creates to kill the virus, because it is easier to measure. If the virus has been in the individual's bloodstream for a sufficient time, it is likely that antibody will have been developed in response to it. Today there are several methods for detecting the antibody.

Blood Tests for the Presence of Antibody

Perhaps the most widely used technique for detecting antibody is the ELISA method, an acronym for Enzyme-Linked Immuno-Sorbent Assay (or EIA, for Enzyme Immunoassay). Developed in 1983 and put into extensive use worldwide by 1985, the ELISA is a rapid and facile method of measurement. During the analysis of an individual's blood sample, a color change on the test signals that antibody is present in the sample—and, by extension, that the virus itself must necessarily have entered the person's bloodstream and may still be present. This is referred to as a "positive" test result and signifies apparent HIV infection. Conversely, if the specified color change does not occur, the antibody is presumably absent, or a "negative" result, usually indicating a lack of infection.

Overall, the ELISA method is sensitive and reliable, being highly effective in the detection of antibody. After an acceptable period of time has elapsed following exposure to the virus, a negative finding on an ELISA is normally regarded as accurate, with no further testing necessary.

In the case of a positive finding, however, the laboratory performs a repeat ELISA on the same blood sample, to double-check the finding. If the second test is also positive, a third test, such as the "Western blot," is typically conducted for final confirmation.

The Western blot technique, like the ELISA, measures the existence of antibody in the blood. By design, however, this method is less sensitive to antibody than the ELISA method; therefore, a more substantial amount of it must be present in a sample before a Western blot analysis will produce a positive finding. After a positive ELISA, a positive Western blot shows that one has been in contact with the virus at some point. In combination, the ELISA–Western blot procedure has an accuracy approaching 100 percent in detecting antibody in a blood sample (1).

Of course, no one test is without its limitations, and the Western blot is no exception. In some cases, and for any number of reasons, complications may arise as the Western blot technique attempts to determine if antibody exists in a given blood sample. In such instances, the result is referred to as indeterminate or inconclusive and may necessitate retesting or the use of additional measures to determine one's HIV status. Indeterminate results that persist through retesting over a period of six months or more are generally considered to indicate a lack of infection.

Despite the impressive sensitivity and utility of antibody tests, an important limitation affects their use. Because several weeks or months are normally required for the immune system to detect the virus and to create antibody to fight it, a measurable level of antibody will not be present during this time. Consequently, a misleading negative test finding may emerge if a person is assessed during the early weeks of the infection. This is a serious problem because it gives an infected person

41

a false sense of security as the virus goes untreated, perhaps being transmitted to others as well.

For this reason, responsible testing sites take special care to ensure that adequate time has elapsed before testing a person for antibody. In some instances, the individual will have a test at their first consultation but be urged to return for retesting several months later, when the immune system will have had sufficient time to respond to the virus.

While this limitation is undeniable, it does not negate the broader value of testing in general, which has gone far in preventing subsequent infection and helping individuals receive prompt treatment to delay the onset of symptoms. Through the development and dissemination of antibody tests in the mid-1980s, we now have extensive screening programs in place for blood donors, thus providing an additional measure of security for our national blood supply. In addition, the relative ease, economy, and versatility of antibody testing has contributed immensely to both large-scale epidemiological research and individual clinical assessment. Most likely, the site that you choose for your own HIV assessment will use antibody tests, since this is by far the most common and expedient form of HIV testing to date.

SALIVA TESTS FOR THE PRESENCE OF ANTIBODY

In addition to the use of blood samples to assess HIV infection, we can now analyze another body fluid—saliva—for the presence of HIV antibodies. A few years ago, researchers found that antibody to HIV could often be detected in the saliva of an infected person, using a sophisticated technique called radioimmunoassay (2). More recently, the ELISA technique described earlier has been modified so that it, too, may detect antibody in saliva, with an accuracy of 98.3 percent having been reported in one particular study (3). While a saliva-based ELISA is relatively sensitive, however, it is still less accurate than a blood-based ELISA. For this reason, the facility at which you seek testing will most likely offer blood tests only.

TESTS FOR THE PRESENCE OF VIRUS

In contrast to "first-generation" antibody tests are those techniques now available to measure characteristics of the virus itself, the best known being the Polymerase Chain Reaction [PCR]. This "second-generation" technique is designed to detect and amplify minute genetic particles of the virus and can therefore effectively locate HIV-infected cells within a very large pool of healthy cells. Because it does not rely on the presence of antibody but looks for the virus itself, this method produces a positive finding soon after the virus enters the body. For these reasons, it is a highly accurate procedure, capable of successfully detecting infection in individuals whose antibody tests initially yield only negative findings. It is also useful for determining whether infection exists in those who receive inconclusive or indeterminate test findings on antibody tests.

The principal limitations of the polymerase chain reaction technique are its extraordinary sensitivity to impurities in samples and its impracticability. Regarding the former, the PCR procedure is highly susceptible to contamination and can easily yield a spurious positive test finding if an impure sample is analyzed. Consequently, rigorous precautions must be followed when preparing and conducting this test.

The test is also impractical because such stringent measures must consistently be practiced to avoid contamination; as a result, it lacks the ease and flexibility of antibody tests. Furthermore, it is an expensive technique and therefore economically prohibitive for widespread application.

HIV Testing Sites

Once you decide to undergo an assessment for HIV infection, you must then choose the kind of testing facility that fits your needs. Many agencies now offer HIV testing, including centers that specialize in the treatment of drug dependence or sexually-transmitted diseases; agencies that offer family planning services; and hospitals and tuberculosis clinics. Three of the most widely used sites today include community AIDS/HIV testing and counseling agencies, the private physician's office, and local health department clinics.

HIV/AIDS TESTING AND COUNSELING CENTERS

Most major cities, and some smaller cities and towns, now maintain free-standing HIV/AIDS service centers designed specifically to address the community's needs. The sole reason for the creation of these agencies, in fact, is to serve the public during the epidemic. Funding is commonly provided by the federal government, with some programs receiving other types of financial support as well. Many services are offered free of charge or for a nominal fee or donation.

Because community testing and counseling centers are designed to serve the entire population, not just the mainstream majority, those who staff them are typically aware of and sensitive to the diverse needs of their clientele; staff tend to be accepting and respectful of alternate life-styles. Also, the staff is usually very well versed in HIV prevention measures as well as current treatments for HIV infection and AIDS. The information provided is timely, relevant, and directly applicable to one's life-style, whatever that may be.

Many agencies offer an array of services, ranging from public education and HIV testing to psychosocial support groups and medical referral services for those who test positive. HIV testing, in particular, normally includes individual counseling before and after the test is conducted to ensure a meaningful and productive assessment experience. In addition, the assessment procedure is most often arranged to give the maximum privacy allowable under state law. It is conducted anonymously in most states, thereby fully protecting the identity of the client.

The only potential drawback found in such specialized service centers is the length of time between the HIV test and the receipt of the test results. In some agencies, due to the high volume of clients seeking assessment—or to the agencies' particular arrangements with laboratories—a few weeks may elapse before the results become available. To the client, of course, the wait may seem interminable. And yet, while a delay may be uncomfortable, it does allow the individual sufficient time to prepare psychologically for the test findings.

In all, as you consider the options available to you, it is important that you appreciate the special value of community HIV/AIDS agencies. These sites provide testing within the context of a supportive counseling relationship, without significant financial expense. Furthermore, should your test findings be positive, this type of agency is well equipped to refer you to appropriate medical, psychological, and legal resources within your community, and possibly to provide certain key services itself. For these reasons, you would be well advised to consider seeking a test at such an agency, since the range and quality of services are often very impressive.

PRIVATE PHYSICIAN'S OFFICE

Another setting in which HIV testing may be conducted is the physician's office. For many, it is common practice to maintain a relationship with a doctor who is aware of one's medical history and, often, with one's broader life circumstances as well. This established, long-term relationship may foster a degree of familiarity, trust, and rapport between doctor and patient not found at other testing sites. If your doctor creates a sense of comfort and security for you, this may be the right choice.

Another advantage may include the relative promptness with which HIV test results are available, sometimes within a matter of days. This reduces the stressful waiting period, and your doctor can begin your medical evaluation and any treatment immediately if the result is positive for HIV. Several valid reasons exist, then, for selecting this setting for an HIV assessment and follow-up care.

Depending on your doctor's experience with HIV and AIDS, however, he or she may not be in the best position to help with all of your needs. Because physicians are trained specifically in the practice of medicine, there may be an accompanying lack of knowledge of other, nonmedical aspects of HIV infection and AIDS. For instance, a physician may be well aware of the clinical manifestations and intricacies of the syndrome yet lack a comprehensive understanding of its broader psychological, sociocultural, and legal ramifications. As a result, your doctor may not be in a suitable position to offer thorough, multidimensional test-related counseling, though providing medical information and treatment.

Similarly, since HIV/AIDS is a new, increasingly specialized area, physicians in other areas of expertise may lack full medical knowledge of the virus, its effects on the immune system, and the efficacies of current treatments for HIV infection and AIDS. Under certain conditions, then, it might not be a realistic expectation for a person to receive both HIV testing and follow-up treatment from his or her personal physician.

A second area of concern involves the privacy of the test findings. Often, the physician feels a professional responsibility to record HIV test results in an individual's medical chart, part of the normal process of maintaining a written chronology of medical care. Unfortunately, the chart may eventually be reviewed by the individual's insurer, and any damaging information might affect future coverage. For this reason, a person should be assessed anonymously when possible, with no written record of the event kept.

In addition, being tested by your doctor means having to pay for the lab work and related services, particularly if you don't want the costs billed to an insurance company. Testing in this setting is therefore costlier than at any other site, despite the fact that the HIV tests used are identical to those at agencies in which assessment is offered free of charge.

When considering being tested by your doctor, you should bear in mind that physicians, like all of us, differ in the extent of their knowledge, social conscience, and emotional sensitivity. They also differ in their HIV testing and reporting practices. For all of these reasons, it is impossible to recommend unequivocally that you seek testing through your physician. Use your own judgment and ask questions if you're not sure.

HEALTH DEPARTMENT CLINICS

Lastly, there are clinics and associated facilities operated by local health departments that provide testing for HIV infection. By and large, such agencies offer easily obtainable, cost-effective services to the public. However, the government, because it finances and operates these sites, may require records of both the client and the HIV test results. Understandably, many individuals are uncomfortable with a government agency's possessing this highly sensitive, potentially damaging information about them, particularly during a period of unprecedented discrimination against carriers of the human immunodeficiency virus. Therefore, if you are considering being tested through the health department, it is advisable that you call the site where you plan to take the test, in advance, to determine if it can be conducted anonymously, or if the use of your name will be necessary. And if you find that your name will indeed be required and you are troubled by this, then pursue testing at another health department site—one that uses anonymous procedures. Of course, make sure that the site you select also provides full counseling before and after the test. If you cannot locate a health department clinic offering these services, consider an alternate testing program, such as an HIV/AIDS testing and counseling center.

Blood Banks

In the past some people have donated blood to blood bank facilities as a way of learning if they were infected with HIV; it is known that these operations routinely screen donations for HIV antibody. However, determining if one is infected in this manner is morally, and in some cases legally, unacceptable. If blood donated by a person early in the course of the infection registered negative (since a sufficient level of antibody would not yet be present), it might be transfused into another, passing on to them the HIV infection. Such an act is therefore potentially dangerous to the population at large and, in some states, is classified as a felony.

If you feel that you may have been in contact with the virus and are in need of a test, choose the kind of testing site that fits your needs and then be tested. The resources are out there for your benefit; use them for your own peace of mind.

Home Test Kits

In recent years, several companies have sought approval from the federal government to market home test kits for HIV infection. To date, the government has refused to permit such kits to be sold to private citizens.

While these tests may possibly provide accurate readings, their use in the home without proper medical supervision and in the absence of effective personal counseling makes them clearly unacceptable. A person should undergo an assessment only at a clinical facility where sufficient counseling is provided before and after the test.

When to Seek an HIV Assessment

Finally, the question of *when* to undergo HIV testing must be resolved. A PCR analysis can be performed very soon after a person has been exposed to the virus and will yield accurate results. Such a test, however, is usually unavailable to the average person. Antibody tests, in contrast, are widely available, but will only yield reliable results when performed several weeks after exposure to HIV (or any point thereafter); this delay allows the immune system adequate time to respond to the virus in a measurable way. In some instances, the body's reaction to the virus will reach a testable level two weeks after exposure to HIV. However, it is usually recommended that a person wait a few more weeks before being tested. Four to twelve weeks are commonly advised.

Researchers have also documented cases in which up to six months have elapsed before an individual has produced a sufficient level of antibody to register on a test. For this reason, it is sometimes recommended that a person undergo a second, follow-up assessment six months after possible exposure to the virus, if the initial test findings are negative.

Many people postpone testing for several months or years after suspected exposure, due to fear or other emotional reactions to the possible outcome. In your own case, you may worry that you harbor the virus yet find yourself reluctant to undergo testing. This is a common, understandable reaction, considering the seri ous nature of HIV infection and its implications. Unfortunately, this response may clearly work against your own best interests, particularly if infection is indeed present.

In most cases it is preferable to be tested relatively soon after contact with the virus. If the results are positive but detected early, the recipient will usually be symptom free and therefore spared the burden of having to cope with the signs of physical illness on top of the bad news. For most people it is arduous enough to contend with the knowledge that one is infected.

In addition, medical intervention, in the form of preventive drugs, can be initiated almost immediately after a positive test result if a medical examination indicates that one's immune system would benefit from the treatment. Research suggests that such medications may be most effective when prescribed early in the course of the infection. Thus, the sooner you are tested, the sooner action can be taken to slow or arrest the infection.

You should bear in mind that many people require a significant amount of time to come to terms with the possibility of infection and to prepare psychologically to undergo HIV testing. Thus, while early assessment is, of course, preferable, and is generally recommended, it is not always possible. The important point is that you be tested if you have reason to believe that you may be infected, even if the infectious event itself transpired many months or years ago.

Before undergoing an assessment, however, it is important that you first familiarize yourself with the central medical, emotional, and legal aspects of the testing process.

51

4

Medical, Legal, and Emotional Considerations in Testing

Most people reach the decision to seek HIV testing only after a period of intense deliberation. This is entirely appropriate and, in fact, the preferred course, since pursuing the test means being prepared to confront the very real possibility of infection. If testing is sought impulsively, without serious forethought, and the findings prove to be positive, the experience may be devastating.

In addition, other problems may arise during or after the assessment if you have an inadequate or distorted understanding of key factors involved in the testing process. Thus, both sufficient psychological preparation and a working knowledge of the test procedures are essential for an optimal assessment experience.

In this chapter, we discuss several pertinent issues involved in the decision to seek or defer HIV testing. The dominant medical issues are presented, followed by an overview of the prevalent legal considerations. We also review the manner in which emotional processes influence an individual's attitude toward assessment. And finally, to further assist you in determining if HIV testing would be beneficial, the chapter concludes with a discussion of four fundamental criteria that should be fulfilled before you proceed with testing.

Medical Issues

An HIV test is performed to determine if an individual is infected with the human immunodeficiency virus. For some, testing may be an indispensable process, while for others it is an unnecessary, time-consuming procedure. Therefore, you should determine if you have good reason to suspect the presence of HIV infection before committing yourself to the assessment.

If you are unsure whether you need testing, review the list provided in Chapter 2 of behaviors and events that put people at risk of infection. You might also contact your local AIDS hotline if you have questions or concerns about your past behaviors and their relationship to infection. (The toll-free telephone numbers for the National AIDS Hotline are provided in Appendix A.)

Another option is to schedule a counseling session at a community HIV/AIDS testing and counseling center before being tested. An HIV counselor would review the various risk factors with you to help determine if testing is warranted.

MEDICAL REASONS FOR SEEKING AN HIV TEST

The principal reason that many individuals decide to undergo assessment is to begin prompt treatment with

53

antiviral medications if the findings reveal that they are infected. Since a positive test result may lead to drug treatment proven to significantly delay the onset of symptoms, a large segment of the population considers this fact instrumental in the decision to seek testing.

Other, more altruistic reasons also exist, including the desire to inform those with whom one has had—or plans to have—intimate contact. Many wish to know their HIV status before entering into new sexual relationships, for instance, so that they might avoid infecting their partners. Many women considering pregnancy also undergo HIV testing to ensure that they will not transmit the infection to the fetus during the pregnancy or at birth. In still other cases, those planning extensive dental or surgical procedures sometimes wish to know if their blood carries the virus so that they can alert the dental or surgical team to the potential risks. These are thoughtful, admirable actions that demonstrate a mature sense of concern and responsibility for the health and well-being of others.

In direct contrast are those who believe that they may well be infected but who nevertheless defer testing. Some may simply believe that HIV tests are inaccurate or unreliable, though this is obviously false. Others think there are no treatments available, so why do anything? Of course, several such therapies are widely attainable. Still, these misconceptions persist within some segments of the population and are clearly harmful when they prevent a person from getting tested.

PARTICIPATION IN MEDICAL RESEARCH

Another misconception involves the idea that getting tested is somehow automatically tied to participation in a scientific study. Since a great amount of research is cur-

rently under way on HIV infection and the potentia̶
ous drugs to treat it, some individuals assume that tl̶
be required to serve as human "guinea pigs" in a re̶ ̶̶ ̶̶ ̶̶
program should their test results prove to be positive. Such
concerns, of course, are completely groundless. Depending
on the circumstances of testing, a person may be invited to
take part in a research study but cannot, in any conceivable
or legal manner, be required to do so. Participation is always at an individual's own discretion and only with his or
her express, written consent.

Legal Issues

In the practice of HIV testing, a dominant legal issue
today involves the necessity of anonymous or confidential testing procedures. On occasion, individuals have
suffered severe penalties for testing positive for the
virus, losing their jobs, their insurance coverage, and
their housing. Furthermore, marked inconsistencies exist
in the federal government's approach to HIV infection
and AIDS. While the public health branch of the government actively encourages testing and even finances HIV
assessment programs, the judicial branch, in sharp contrast, offers only limited, inconsistent legal protection
for those who test positive. Accordingly, many individuals voice concerns about the protection of their identities during the assessment process. Such concerns are
legitimate and merit serious consideration.

ANONYMOUS VERSUS CONFIDENTIAL TESTING

To protect your privacy, you should only have an
HIV test at an agency that guarantees anonymity or

confidentiality throughout the assessment process. An agency's policy and practices may be determined in advance simply by asking.

In *anonymous* testing procedures, one's name is never known or recorded by the agency. Instead, a code number or other form of nonpersonal, untraceable identification is assigned to the person and used throughout the assessment process. Most community HIV/AIDS testing and counseling agencies operate in this fashion, when permissible under state law.

By comparison, *confidential* testing does involve the use of one's name as well as certain demographic information in some instances. The individual's identity and test findings are normally protected from disclosure to other sources, however, unless the test recipient first consents to their release. Medical facilities, including physicians in private practice, routinely use confidential procedures.

MANDATORY TESTING

There are some instances in which an individual may be asked to undergo mandatory testing, a controversial issue. At the present time, several major insurance companies require an applicant for health or life insurance to undergo an HIV test before they will issue a policy. If the applicant tests positive, coverage will almost certainly be limited or denied. Similarly, applicants to the U.S. military are required to undergo HIV testing and, if infected, are refused entry into the service. Furthermore, those already in the military are now being tested and, if found to be HIV-positive, are reassigned within the military system.

Should you find yourself facing mandatory assessment, it might be advisable for you to seek an anonymous test at a community testing center to find out your HIV status in advance. If you test positive, it may well be to your advantage to cancel the mandatory assessment session. In this way, you will be able to preserve and protect your privacy.

In the event that you are already covered by a health insurance policy, you should be aware that your HIV status may still become known to your insurer. While confidential practices normally protect your medical records from outside scrutiny, your insurance company does have access to them, a right you usually agree to as a condition of their coverage. Consequently, should you decide to seek testing through your private physician, as discussed in Chapter 3, the findings may be placed in your medical record and eventually reviewed by your insurance company. And this may prove detrimental.

To sidestep such a potentially awkward situation, you should inquire about your doctor's reporting policy prior to undergoing the test. Many physicians today are sensitive to the possibility of discrimination against HIV-positive individuals and thus do not record such test findings in their patients' medical charts. Other practitioners, in contrast, do feel obliged by medical ethics to document the findings. If your physician plans to record your HIV test findings, you might consider seeking anonymous testing at a community HIV/AIDS testing and counseling center as an alternative, particularly if you anticipate a positive test.

REPORTING LAWS

Twenty-one states currently require that an individual's name and HIV test results be reported to the local or state health department. There, the information is purportedly held in strict confidence and is used only to monitor the epidemic. An additional twelve states require the reporting of HIV test results but not the names of those who receive them. In this way, the state has the capacity to track the number and locations of new infections, yet in a manner that protects the identities of the test recipients themselves. And in seventeen states and the District of Columbia, neither names nor findings are reported. A complete list of reporting practices, by state, is provided in Appendix B.

Many citizens would not seek an HIV assessment if they knew that their names and test findings would be forwarded to a government health department, and it is for this reason that many states do not require the reporting of such information. Further, even those that do mandate the reporting of names sometimes provide the means by which a person may undergo anonymous testing.

Before your own assessment, you might wish to contact an AIDS hotline, public health department, or other resource to determine if your state requires the reporting of your name and HIV test results to the health department. If you do live in one of those states, you might inquire into possible ways to circumvent the requirement. If your anonymity is not assured by laws in your own state, you might consider seeking an HIV assessment in a neighboring state where anonymous testing is legal. In some cases, people use assumed names during the assessment process to protect their true identities.

A related legal matter that is of concern for intravenous drug users and those in the sex industry, in particular, involves the fear that their illicit activities will be discovered and lead to prosecution. In actuality, the specific manner in which one may have become infected remains confidential in virtually all test settings, even in government clinics, and therefore an individual is not normally reported to the authorities for an illegal act that may have caused the contraction of the virus. When such information is sought from the client about the source of infection, it is for the mapping of evolving epidemiological trends; that is, the material is collected to help us better understand the ways in which the virus is being spread, and the segments of the population into which it is reaching. Such information is indispensable for the design and implementation of public health programs to fight the epidemic. Since these researchers are not concerned with the legality of a particular lifestyle, however, there is no reason to fear that information given in the assessment process will have legal repercussions.

Special Concerns of Minorities

Finally, a significant problem sometimes exists within Hispanic and African-American groups who feel themselves victimized and discriminated against by the American medical establishment. This legacy of anger, mistrust, and rejection is reportedly widespread. Specifically, they feel that their medical care has historically been substandard and that they have been the victims of exploitation. Accordingly, Hispanic and African-American people sometimes shun HIV testing, viewing it as yet another way in which they might be further stigmatized, ostracized, or manipulated by the mainstream medical community.

Yet these people should realize that HIV testing is

clearly to their own advantage. Often, it can be performed in a variety of settings, including neighborhood clinics staffed by members of their own subculture.

Another concern involves same-sex relationships within the Hispanic and African-American subcultures, where overt male homosexuality has traditionally been bitterly denounced. As a result, many homosexual and bisexual men are understandably reluctant to undergo HIV testing for fear that their sexual preferences will become known in their communities. These gentlemen should realize, however, that the nature of their sexual lives and practices will be protected from public disclosure when HIV testing is conducted in a setting that adheres to anonymous or confidential testing procedures.

Emotional Issues

Psychological influences also play a prominent role in the decision to seek an HIV test. In some instances, people feel compelled to be tested, while different emotional factors may prevent others from proceeding with an assessment. It is therefore important to recognize the power of psychological influences.

PSYCHOLOGICAL REASONS FOR SEEKING AN HIV TEST

One fundamental reason people seek out HIV testing is to restore a sense of stability and peace of mind; to determine if they are infected with the virus, rather than live with nagging doubt and uncertainty. To many people, knowing definitely whether they have HIV is far preferable to uncertainty about their health, medical future, and chance of infecting others.

An individual may also seek testing within the context of a larger, more pervasive trend toward self-evaluation and change. As one approaches a critical period in life, a need to examine, evaluate, and modify one's way of life may emerge. Such a period may occur, for instance, following the dissolution of a long-term romantic relationship or at the beginning of a new one; following the decision to openly declare and explore one's homosexual or bisexual feelings; after an encounter with potentially serious illness or a brush with mortality; or as a result of other major life events that force an individual to take stock of his or her overall situation. And an important aspect of this process may be a review of health concerns to determine if change is needed and, if so, the direction of such change. In this sense, an HIV test may lead to substantive life-style modification.

In the midst of such self-evaluation and change, a positive HIV test often spurs the individual to begin treatment for the infection and may radically influence his or her manner of living to promote health, longevity, and quality of life. A negative test often accomplishes the same thing, with this "clean bill of health" seen as an opportunity to approach life with a renewed sense of purpose leading to new goals and commitments. In either case, the test findings have served as a catalyst for change.

Of course, other psychological factors may complicate the decision to seek an assessment. Many well-adjusted individuals who face the prospect of HIV testing procrastinate, at least temporarily. They genuinely intend to undergo testing but repeatedly postpone or otherwise delay the appointment. This tendency is a sign of unresolved issues on some level, such as the interference of fears and anxieties. It follows, then, that by lifting these underlying emotional blocks, the impasse will dissolve and one will be able to proceed with the assessment.

If you find yourself procrastinating, you should seek out the hidden concerns that may be preventing you from continuing with the assessment. If you are unable to identify such reasons, or if you continue to procrastinate, a counselor can often help you to understand and remove the resistance to testing.

Of course, many people avoid testing simply out of the fear of being unable to cope with a positive test finding—the fear that emotional trauma will ensue. It is entirely possible that a person will initially have difficulty coming to terms with a positive finding, although most who do get tested eventually adjust satisfactorily. Still, it is counterproductive to encourage an emotionally fragile individual to undergo HIV testing when a positive finding could conceivably tax the person's mental and physical resources beyond their limits. In such a case, the goal of testing would be largely defeated.

A related emotional process that sometimes causes a person to refrain from being tested is referred to as the "white coat syndrome"—a profound fear of medical practices and procedures. A person with such a fear is apprehensive about virtually all aspects of the medical experience out of an irrational belief that some indefinable yet utterly horrendous event awaits him or her at a clinical facility. Emotionally paralyzed by this phobia, the person will accept medical attention only when circumstances demand it, such as during a mandatory pre-employment physical examination or upon developing an undeniably serious illness. In the case of HIV testing, the individual may clearly understand the need for it but simply be immobilized by anxiety and unable to proceed with the assessment.

If you find yourself experiencing any of these difficulties, you would probably benefit from a comprehensive pretest counseling session with an HIV counselor. With the facts at hand and a supportive counselor at your side, you can better gauge your ability to cope with the potential test results, while also easing any irrational anxieties you might harbor. In fact, a principal reason that most HIV testing agencies recommend or require counseling prior to the blood test is to address these matters. If, for some reason, you are uncomfortable discussing your difficulties at an HIV testing and counseling center or don't have access to one, you might arrange a meeting with a private therapist or physician and use this professional as a support source throughout the testing process.

Criteria for Seeking an HIV Test

Obviously, the decision to have an HIV assessment is not a simple one, and it does require deep thought about your goals and fears. Being tested for HIV infection is a critical, irreversible act, and you must weigh all aspects of the test and its implications before you reach a final decision. Paradoxically, it helps to remember that HIV testing, although potentially beneficial to hundreds of thousands of people, may not be appropriate for everyone. And even when assessment is advisable, its timing is an important consideration. You have to be ready physically, mentally, and emotionally. To help in determining if you should undergo such a test, four fundamental criteria should be met before you proceed with the assessment process.

First, you should be relatively certain that you may have been in contact with the virus. If you are unsure, review Chapter 2 and/or contact an AIDS hotline or similar resource to get clear-eyed help in examining your level of risk. If there is any chance of HIV contact in your history, then consider getting tested.

Second, you should seek an HIV assessment only at a facility that subscribes to anonymous, or at least confidential, testing procedures; otherwise, your privacy may be compromised because of widespread discrimination. Whether you select anonymous or confidential testing, the salient point is that strict safeguards for your privacy be in place throughout the assessment.

Third, you should be emotionally prepared to cope with a positive test result. If you are currently facing a number of stressful life events, this may not be the best time to seek testing; perhaps it should be delayed until you have reduced these pressures or have developed a sufficient support network to help you cope with the situation. Likewise, if you tend to be emotionally fragile, have a history of moodiness or suicidal tendencies, or have other reasons to doubt your ability to contend with a positive test finding, then you might consider establishing a relationship with an HIV counselor, psychotherapist, pastoral counselor, or other professional who can provide assistance and support during assessment.

And finally, medical services should be available following testing. In the event that your findings indicate the presence of infection. Although the facility at which you undergo the test may not be equipped to furnish these services directly, it should nevertheless be in a position to refer you to medical resources in your community. In this way, the assessment phase can proceed quickly and easily to treatment.

5

Negative Test Results and Inconclusive Test Results

A negative finding on an antibody test ordinarily denotes the absence of infection, and people usually meet such news with overwhelming relief, even exhilaration. In fact, interpreting such a finding as unequivocal good news may be hasty and premature, since a negative test result can have diverse meanings depending on various factors.

In this chapter, we review the various interpretations of negative findings, as well as the adaptive and maladaptive behavioral reactions that sometimes accompany them. We also consider the significance of an inconclusive, or indeterminate, test finding. In all, the discussion should provide you with a more complete understanding of these types of test results—information that could prove useful to you.

Negative Test Results

In the majority of cases, a negative finding on an HIV antibody test means that a person is free from infection. Assuming that the individual was not at an inordinately high risk for infection and that sufficient time was allowed for the immune system to develop antibody prior to testing, the finding is probably accurate. And because the test result is, in all likelihood, valid, further testing is usually unnecessary.

Of course, under certain circumstances the meaning of a negative finding may be somewhat less definite. For instance, a negative result will occur if antibody testing is conducted too early in the course of the infection, before the immune system has had adequate time to produce a measurable level of antibody. As we discussed in Chapter 3, it typically requires six to twelve weeks following infection with the virus for antibody to be detectable, although it has been known to take up to six months. Sufficient time must therefore elapse before an assessment is conducted.

Oddly, another occasion when misleading negative findings may occur is during the advanced stages of AIDS. It does happen that, well into the disease process, the immune system becomes depleted of antibody as a consequence of its long-term struggle against the virus. A test finding will therefore register negative, despite the presence of widespread HIV infection.

Other medical conditions—unrelated to AIDS—also exist that may produce false-negative findings in HIV antibody tests. These include the presence of a malignancy, blood replacement (transfusion), bone marrow transplantation, and immunosuppressive treatment (1).

And finally, a rather unlikely event that may yield an

invalid negative finding is a mistake at the facility that processes the blood test, a technical or clerical error in the lab. The chances of this happening, though, are quite remote, since clinical facilities tend to be meticulous in their clinical and record-keeping practices.

In regard to those specialized methods that measure elements of the virus itself, such as PCR analysis, these techniques yield results soon after a person's contact with the virus and tend to be highly accurate. Accordingly, a negative result on a measure of this type may be confidently accepted as indicating freedom from infection, with no further corroboration necessary. Unfortunately, PCR is both unwieldy and expensive, and thus not often available for normal, routine testing.

Emotional Reactions to Negative Test Results

The most common response to a negative test finding is immense relief and a sense of liberation and release. Often the person feels elated and exuberant or has profound feelings of humility and gratitude. The reaction is pleasant, personally meaningful, and deeply restorative.

It is not unusual for a person to experience the negative test results as a symbolic reprieve and to use the event as a springboard for substantive behavioral change. For someone wishing to begin a new love relationship, for example, the news that he or she is infection-free brings confidence and reassurance that the virus will not be passed to the partner. For the couple desiring children, negative findings in both persons permit them to begin their family without worry about their children's health. For the individual having symptoms suggestive of AIDS, the test result may signal the presence of another type of illness and point to a definitive diagnosis in a different direction. In several ways, then, a person may be liberated or at least substantially redirected by a negative test result.

A rather vivid example of all of this is provided by Alex, a young man I counseled when he came in for HIV testing at the metropolitan testing agency where I worked. A junior at a local university, Alex had been experiencing fever, swollen glands, sore throat, and fatigue and was intensely concerned that his symptoms might be AIDS-related. So distraught was he, in fact, that his personal relationships were becoming strained, and his academic performance was sharply declining.

Apparently, Alex had become deeply preoccupied with his condition and had lost interest in most other activities—a common reaction to the fear of HIV infection. He explained that, among other problems, he seemed to be developing severe anxiety regarding sex, including a marked fear that he might pass or had already passed the infection to the woman he was dating. Not surprisingly, their relationship was in turmoil because of these sudden, sweeping changes in Alex's mood and behavior. Evidently, he was uncomfortable discussing his worries about HIV infection with his girlfriend. He also told me that he was considering temporarily withdrawing from college, solely due to the impact that these HIV-related concerns were having on his life and academic abilities.

Immediately before coming to us he had had a physical examination through his personal physician, at which point various tests were conducted to determine the nature of his symptoms. He added that he was seeking an HIV assessment from our agency because our tests were conducted anonymously.

Alex had, he said, engaged in some risky sexual behavior during his first semester of college, when he had occasionally participated in recreational sex with another male student. These experiences occurred with his roommate in the dormitory and, except for a cursory exploration of oral sex, consisted exclusively of mutual masturbation. When his roommate transferred to another college, the contact ceased. His subsequent encounters had been with three different women and involved oral and vaginal intercourse. No other sexual experiences or potentially risky activities were noted in Alex's history.

His doctor's tests had revealed, just prior to his HIV results, that Alex had the Epstein-Barr virus, otherwise known as innocuous infectious mononucleosis. Fortunately, mononucleosis is a relatively common, treatable illness. And while the presence of the Epstein-Barr virus did not, in itself, preclude the existence of HIV infection, it would nevertheless be a very likely explanation for his symptoms in the absence of HIV.

On the HIV antibody test, Alex tested negative. When I told him about these results, he became very emotional; his sense of relief was strong and clearly visible. As his composure returned, he discussed the persistent stress he had endured while waiting for the findings to arrive and the enormous amount of time he had spent contemplating his situation. In all, Alex appeared to have made sensible, well-organized plans in anticipation of either positive or negative test results.

Since the findings were negative, he decided to remain in school and work hard to catch up academically. He added that he would now consider applying to graduate school as well—an issue about which he had apparently felt some ambivalence in the past. Furthermore, Alex felt free to explain his recent behavior changes to his girlfriend, and conveyed his belief that she would be sympathetic. He expressed his hope of visiting his family in the near future, stating that he felt much closer to them now, even though none of his family members had been aware of his recent difficulties. In all, then, this experience appeared to help clarify and enhance Alex's life and future. It also illustrates the profound energy and direction that may emerge from a negative test finding.

In contrast to such a productive reaction, sometimes people misinterpret a negative result. For instance, people can look on it as proof that they are immune to the virus; that if their previous risky behavior has not given them HIV, then some sort of constitutional factor must be protecting them against infection. Of course, looking on themselves in this light obviates the need to take personal responsibility to practice precautions and avoid further risky behavior, a very negative attitude that can be dangerous to them and to others. In reality, the bulk of currently available research suggests that most everyone is potentially vulnerable to HIV infection. If an individual who has engaged in unsafe practices has not contracted it, the person has simply been very fortunate. If he or she persists, infection may yet occur. No one is invincible.

In still other cases, a person may experience such profound relief at receiving a negative test finding that they rush, in their euphoria, to gratify those impulses that would normally be inhibited or safely channeled. Thus, while in the midst of celebrating a negative finding, a person may unwittingly move directly into the path of the virus itself; ironic, considering that one is presumably responding to the absence of infection.

In contrast are those who have no desire to celebrate their good fortune; they feel sad, guilty, confused, even apologetic for testing negative. Referred to as "survivor guilt," this unpleasant emotional response may emerge when one's lover, spouse, or close friend tests HIV-positive, leaving the person who tests negative feeling ashamed or unworthy of being healthy. Even when one is not intimately involved with an HIV-positive person, he or she may still identify with a group at increased risk, such as with the gay community, and feel estranged or excluded from the community upon receiving a negative test result. These feelings of personal unworthiness—of not "deserving" freedom from infection—are more likely to haunt a person who is by nature guilt-prone or who suffers from chronic low self-esteem, but the reaction may still occur in virtually anyone.

In some instances, survivor guilt lifts spontaneously after a short time. In other instances, such emotions motivate an individual to act on behalf of those who *are* infected, to become a volunteer in an AIDS service organization or an activist for an AIDS-related issue. Unfortunately, survivor guilt persists in some people regardless of any action they take. If remorse and sadness do not subside, professional counseling and/or a support group for partners or family members of HIV-positive individuals is advisable.

Finally, there is the exceptional individual who refuses to believe or accept a negative test finding as valid. Even when the person's life-style is characterized by very few risk factors, no symptoms of illness, and negative HIV test findings, this person remains staunchly convinced that he or she is infected and is destined to develop AIDS. In cases of this sort, professional intervention may be necessary before the person is able to discard the distorted belief and accept the reality of the negative test findings.

Inconclusive or Indeterminate Test Results

Occasionally, a Western blot analysis or similar test can neither confirm nor deny the presence of antibody in a blood sample, and the finding is therefore classified as "inconclusive" or "indeterminate." This happens for several reasons.

In some cases, a very small amount of antibody may be present in the bloodstream but in a quantity insufficient to register markedly on the test. In other cases, unique properties of the blood itself—factors having nothing whatsoever to do with HIV infection—may interfere with the analysis and obscure the findings. And finally, technical problems or accidents in the laboratory may produce inconclusive or indeterminate results.

Normally, the test is simply repeated, although periodic retesting on several occasions is sometimes necessary before an inconclusive finding can be satisfactorily clarified. If an individual continues to receive indeterminate test results for six months or longer, the person is usually considered to be negative for HIV infection.

Obviously, an indeterminate test result can be an emotionally trying experience. For those having difficulty coping with uncertainty or ambiguity, the inconclusive test is a distinct emotional challenge. It is essential to remember, however, that there are numerous reasons for an indeterminate test result and that conclusions cannot be drawn until definitive information becomes available.

If you test inconclusively, don't panic. Work closely

with your HIV counselor or physician to arrange re-testing or additional procedures. Keep a rational perspective on the situation and ask your counselor for support in maintaining a manageable anxiety level. As your physician or counselor will tell you, the finding essentially reveals nothing about your HIV status. Ultimately, with persistence and patience, you will learn whether or not you are free of HIV infection.

6

Coping with Positive Test Results

Upon receiving a positive test finding, a person usually experiences many conflicting and disturbing emotional reactions, which depend, of course, on one's personality, current life circumstances, and knowledge of the human immunodeficiency virus and its treatment. To the testing situation, then, each person brings a distinct assortment of fears, needs, hopes, and beliefs, and it is largely through the interplay of these factors that an individual's emotional response is determined and shaped. Of course, the reaction may also be colored by external considerations, such as marital, social, occupational, and financial concerns.

Because these contributing factors tend to be diverse, it is somewhat difficult to predict how you will respond if you test positive; clearly, reactions tend to be unique.

Certain responses do appear to be more common than

others, however, and in this chapter we will begin by examining the thoughts and feelings you may experience and review those actions that may help ease emotional distress. We will also discuss the process many infected individuals go through to attain some kind of philosophical understanding of the infection, the ways people move toward a reconciliation with, and acceptance of, the condition. The chapter concludes with an overview of the productive life orientation that can emerge from a successful adjustment to the HIV-positive state.

Emotional Reactions

DENIAL OF REALITY

When you receive positive test results, your first reaction may well be one of astonishment, combined with an inability to accept the reality of the findings. Even if you have anticipated testing positive, you may still find yourself stunned or dazed at this confirmation, and you may experience a temporarily diminished capacity to engage in meaningful thought or emotion. Such a condition is harmless, however, as well as brief, usually lasting only a few minutes in most instances.

Considered to be an adaptive response, this fleeting emotional condition protects you from being completely incapacitated by the unpleasant news. By numbing your feelings, it decreases the sense of vulnerability and discomfort you might otherwise experience, while also allowing time for additional psychological defenses to come into play. As a result, you will be better equipped to cope as this state of emotional numbness dissipates.

You may then experience a second reaction, called "denial," a protective emotional device, whereby an individual refuses to accept or attempts to gain a sense of distance from the reality of a situation. This is because that reality is too painful to allow into consciousness.

Such a process may be occurring, if, for instance, you find yourself questioning the accuracy of the HIV test or entertaining the possibility of having accidentally received another person's test findings. You may doubt, too, the competence of the laboratory or the counselor or technician who reported the test results to you. You may even ask for retesting to be certain that the results are valid. Though the motive may be denial on your part, a confirmatory test is always advisable, particularly if the findings were based on a single test.

In most people, the denial process gradually diminishes, giving way to higher-level coping mechanisms. There are occasions, however, when this reaction persists, with the individual permanently failing to acknowledge the positive test findings. As a result, he or she may continue to live as if completely healthy, thereby inadvertently spreading the virus to others. Hopefully, you will pass through the denial phase satisfactorily, accept the reality of the positive finding, and proceed to more adaptive forms of coping with the test results.

Gradually, as you emerge from this initial period of emotional overload, you will begin to confront the actual meaning of the HIV infection itself. This confrontational process is difficult and turbulent. You may experience unpleasant extremes of fear, sadness, and the anticipation of loss. Despite the discomfort, however, such responses are natural, healthy, and essential elements of adjusting and therefore, in themselves, should not be a cause for alarm.

FEAR AND ANTICIPATED LOSS

The fear and anxiety that often accompany a positive finding can be so intense that an individual will go to remarkable lengths to push away, or even escape, these feelings. In most cases, though, your natural coping resources, in conjunction with the passage of time, serve to lessen the tumultuous feelings to a considerable degree, until you eventually become able to reflect on and discuss the infection without anxiety or distress.

The reason for this deep apprehension is related in large part to the way a person interprets the meaning of a positive test result. Sometimes an individual equates HIV infection with AIDS, and AIDS with death. As a result, the person feels powerless, even doomed. In reality, HIV infection is not all that awesome and can now be slowed or arrested for protracted periods of time with proper medication. Indeed, for the average individual infected with the virus, several years elapse before noticeable symptoms appear, symptoms for which we now have an arsenal of therapies more effective than those of the past. And yet the initial expectation in a substantial number of cases is that of immediate, incapacitating illness or demise and is accompanied by intense fear and panic.

Being armed with the right facts can go a long way to forestall such a response. A positive finding is not synonymous with immediate illness or mortality but only means that your chances of eventually developing certain types of illness are increased. We have made remarkable strides medically since the virus first permeated our society, and these advancements have significantly altered the course of the syndrome in a large number of cases. Furthermore, all indications are that additional breakthroughs are forthcoming, if not around the corner.

Blending with this concern over possible illness may be feelings of loss, despair, and depression. Particularly if you are a young or middle-aged adult, the prospect of terminal illness, regardless of its immediate manifestation, may be exceedingly difficult to accept. You may begin to anticipate losses relevant to young or middle-aged individuals, such as a feared disruption or loss of your college education or career, inability to fulfill parental obligations, or loss of physical attractiveness and youthful appeal. You may also fear that your spouse, lover, family, or friends will abandon or ostracize you, or that your illness will tear you away from them and their love. Being infected with HIV may even trigger a loss of self-respect and self-esteem, because the infection is so often associated with socially unacceptable sexual or drug practices. The sheer number of potential losses, then, can be staggering. Fortunately, it is most common that a person becomes concerned with only one or two such potential losses and attempts to cope with them specifically.

Through contemplation, education, and the healing effects of time itself, you will eventually adopt a different view of your situation. Infected individuals frequently come to realize that the anticipated losses that earlier seemed so vivid, immediate, and imminent may actually not occur for several years, if ever. They discover, too, that those with whom they share especially close, intimate relationships—spouses or long-term lovers—do not necessarily shun or reject them for testing positive but sometimes display an unexpected degree of kindness, nurturance, and loyalty. And in most instances, it appears that HIV-positive individuals choose to continue their educations and careers, while making singular efforts to preserve or enhance their health and well-being. Therefore, as you adjust to the HIV infection, you, too, will find your perspective changing to a more productive and life-affirming one, and your initial fears will give way to a more realistic long-term perspective on the future.

As you dwell on the potential losses described earlier, however, feelings of depression may become quite pronounced and you may find yourself temporarily withdrawing from social interaction. This is entirely normal and provides you with the solitude necessary to work through important personal issues. This emotional state usually engenders feelings of sadness, discouragement, and hopelessness, sometimes accompanied by remorse or regret over past actions. These are ordinary characteristics of a depressed condition and, while unpleasant to experience, are considered a natural and necessary part of adjusting to the awareness of HIV infection.

It is possible, though, that you may enter into a depressed condition without experiencing these usual symptoms of depression. The signs may instead be more subtle and indirect; they may include increased irritability, hostility, and argumentativeness, or sudden increases in your activity level or number of outside social or career involvements. You may also find yourself prone to impulsive, poorly planned changes in significant areas of your life, such as making a sudden, hasty decision to relocate or initiating sweeping changes in your relationships or career. Other symptoms may include a diminished attention span, difficulty concentrating, temporarily decreased memory capacity, or a marked preoccupation with HIV-related issues.

You should also know that there are features of a depressive reaction that you might mistake for symptoms of AIDS itself: Loss of appetite (resulting in weight loss), changes in sleep patterns (resulting in fatigue), and other stress-related symptoms. It sometimes happens that an infected person believes such changes to signal the onset of AIDS, thus triggering even more fear, anxiety, and depression, and further undermining the person's physical and emotional well-being. It is for this reason that educational and counseling resources must be readily available for all those infected. Coping with the genuine aspects of the condition can be quite taxing at times, without the added burden and unnecessary stress created by misconceptions and misunderstandings.

I witnessed the effects that stress and depression may have on a person's physical functioning while helping Emily, a woman who contracted the virus from a tainted blood transfusion. Emily told me that she'd had to have emergency surgery requiring a blood transfusion after sustaining injuries in an automobile accident. Following her recovery and discharge from the hospital, a hospital representative called and informed her that the transfusion she had received may have been impure, and they advised testing for HIV infection. Emily did seek an HIV assessment, and her test was positive.

Until that time, she had felt well physically, with no symptoms of illness. But after receiving the results, Emily became depressed and despondent, withdrawing from most social activities. The only people she told of her infection were her husband and mother, both of whom also became distressed by the situation; nevertheless, they were remarkably supportive.

A few weeks later, Emily appeared at our HIV testing agency, told us that she was HIV-positive and that she had since developed serious concerns that she needed to discuss with a counselor. When I saw her a few moments later, she seemed tense, nervous, and fearful. Her face was pale and drawn, and she looked exhausted. As our discussion progressed, it became evident that her emotions were intense and very close to the surface; she was distraught and became tearful with little provocation.

In desperate tones, Emily confided her fear that she was already experiencing symptoms of AIDS. She reported that in recent weeks her appetite had lessened, she had lost weight, and she felt "slowed down" and tired much of the time. She had developed a mild respiratory infection, too, and feared that this illness might mark the beginning of AIDS-related Pneumocystis pneumonia. In fact, it was this respiratory illness that ultimately prompted her visit to our agency. During our discussion, Emily repeatedly asked if her symptoms were indicative of AIDS, as well as requesting the names of medical facilities where she could get effective treatment for the condition.

After hearing her concerns, I recommended that she pursue her medical questions with her personal physician, or with a doctor from our agency's listing of AIDS specialists in the city. I also enrolled her in one of our support groups.

Emily followed these suggestions and underwent a thorough medical examination. Her health was found to be satisfactory. Except for a common and relatively harmless respiratory infection, which was quickly eradicated with antibiotics, she displayed no symptoms of illness. Instead, her symptoms appeared to stem from the feelings of depression she was experiencing in response to the positive test findings.

During her subsequent involvement in the support group, Emily discussed her concerns openly, and this provided a much-needed emotional outlet and helped her organize her thoughts and restructure her life. Consequently, her appetite improved, as did her ability to sleep at night. Her energy level also increased, while the problems with fatigue dissipated. Nevertheless, Emily still had the occasional tendency to become anxious at innocuous physical symptoms like a skin irritation or sore throat—a tendency very familiar to those infected with HIV. Over the course of time, however, she became increasingly adept at responding in a reasonable manner to such everyday medical problems.

In your own life, as you adjust to the HIV condition, feelings of hopelessness and despondency will likely diminish at some point, and the depression will lift. Your energy level will increase, your mood will return to normal and, although it will probably have changed in some respects, your view of life will again most likely become productive. If the depression proves to be especially intense or tenacious, however, and does not abate within a few days or weeks, you should consider seeking psychological counseling. This may entail psychotherapy, time-limited counseling, behavior therapy, or supportive group intervention, all of which can be accomplished on an outpatient basis with assurances of confidentiality. In a few cases, effective treatment may also include the temporary use of antidepressant medication in concert with counseling or therapy.

An extreme degree of depression may temporarily cloud your outlook and diminish the ability to make sound decisions, especially if you're also coping with feelings of panic, anxiety, and fear. For instance, a certain percentage of individuals, upon learning of their positive HIV status, consider ending their lives. Of course, most do not actually pursue this notion further, but the option does at least occur to them, reflecting their striking fear and initial confusion. As a person gains a greater sense of emotional control, however, these ideas typically fade, and the individual once again becomes able to think clearly and rationally and to function purposefully.

If you should find yourself feeling anxious, frightened, or dejected to this degree, try to organize your time to be around others until the urge to end your life diminishes. Call a friend or visit with others until your feelings of emotional control and stability return. Also, contacting a local crisis intervention service, suicide hotline, or AIDS hotline can be extremely helpful, since a telephone counselor can provide you with emotional support and guidance and serve as a source of reason and objectivity while you are experiencing inner turmoil. Brief, supportive therapy can also help you contend with the upset and may further guide you into healthier methods of coping with HIV positivity in the future. Support groups, particularly those for individuals with HIV infection, can be very valuable as well, since the group's members will likely share your experiences, concerns, and needs and therefore be capable of genuine understanding. The important point is that you not hesitate in seeking assistance to stabilize your mental state and calm the emotional storm. Resources are available and should be used.

Most often, an infected person does not react so strongly as to require some of the types of intervention described here. But even those who are able to cope effectively with their feelings may find support groups and other growth-enhancement strategies quite useful. Like other life crises, HIV positivity, emotionally unpleasant though it may be, may serve as a catalyst for inner growth and development.

ASSOCIATED EMOTIONAL REACTIONS

As you cope with a positive test finding, you may find yourself experiencing other types of reactions besides or in addition to those already described. Although they do not occur in every individual, there are some responses that occur frequently enough to warrant discussion.

The first involves marked feelings of frustration and anger. Obviously, to be confronted with a potentially serious illness for which there is, as yet, no cure may be deeply frustrating. As a result, feelings of futility and exasperation may emerge abruptly and intensely, expressing themselves in a variety of ways. It is not unusual, for instance, for such hostility to compel an individual to place blame for the viral condition on a specific source.

Some infected people turn the focus inward, blaming themselves for having become infected with the virus even when their personal histories suggest they were clearly unaware of the risks involved at the time of infection. Others may be inclined to direct their hostility toward others, assigning blame to a particular person from whom the virus may have been contracted. Feelings of anger and resentment aimed at the government and the medical establishment for alleged irresponsibility and negligence during the epidemic are also common. Indeed, most observers agree that the government has failed on numerous occasions to act rapidly and decisively during this profound public health crisis, with terrible effects for the public at large.

Despite its initial shortcomings, the medical community has actually made remarkable strides in its counterattack on the virus in the decade since the epidemic began. Nevertheless, many infected individuals and collectives of AIDS patients continue to bombard the medical establishment with an enormous amount of rage. And while a certain amount of anger may be warranted in specific cases, in other instances it is almost certainly a misdirected expression of the infected person's fear and frustration at harboring a potentially lethal virus.

The target of one's anger serves as an outlet, a tangible target toward which one may channel feelings of aggression. Blaming oneself, however, tends to be counterproductive, impeding adjustment to the condition by reducing feelings of self-worth and promoting depression. Directing anger toward institutions, such as the medical establishment, may likewise work against a person's best interests, especially if it prevents or delays the individual's seeking treatment, because this ultimately undermines their physical well-being.

Should you find yourself feeling marked frustration, hostility, or resentment, you might reduce your anger by taking stronger action to preserve your health and fitness. By assuming greater responsibility for maintaining, and even improving, your immune system, you will experience a stronger sense of control, and your vulnerability and frustration will lessen. Of course, if you feel that your hostility is warranted and wish to express it, then you should do so in a socially responsible, constructive manner, and in a way that will not interfere with or otherwise jeopardize your physical health or medical treatment.

Another reaction that sometimes occurs involves the effect of HIV-positivity on self-image and self-respect. To some, being infected with HIV means they are "tainted" in some manner. Consequently, they no longer identify with or enjoy their bodies and may become extremely reluctant to kiss, embrace, or even touch others, although they understand that to do so is harmless. This reaction seems due in large part to the fact that the virus can be spread through certain forms of sexual contact and through illicit drug use—activities considered unacceptable by some infected persons.

If you feel affected by HIV in this way, you should bear in mind that the infectious agent is a virus, and virtually everyone has suffered from a viral infection at some point in their lives. In the case of HIV, the agent is simply much more resistant than others to which we have been exposed. By viewing the condition as a medical entity, rather than as a reflection of your general worth as a person, you will assume a more realistic perspective and will move forward in your emotional adjustment.

The Quest for Meaning

As you continue to cope with the HIV condition, you may find yourself increasingly drawn toward reflection and self-evaluation, and this may eventually give rise to substantial personal change. This is very common in infected individuals and may even be considered a prominent feature of the adjustment process. Often, these inclinations seem to emerge in the depressive phase of the coping process, during which you may feel the need to embark on an emotional or spiritual journey in an effort to better understand why you became infected. Such a quest, if successful, can lead not only to a more complete reconciliation with the HIV infection, but to a richer, deeper, and more intense appreciation of the process of life itself.

When you learn that you harbor the human immunodeficiency virus, your view of the world as a predictable and secure haven may vanish, replaced instead by a marked sense of vulnerability to forces beyond your personal control. You may experience a heightened awareness of the power and capriciousness of nature, as well as your own fragility in the face of it. Understandably, this can be rather unsettling, and you may feel a pressing need to restore a sense of security, control, and certainty to your life. Thus, by having your views thrown into doubt through the turmoil of infection, you may find it necessary to reexamine your earlier ideas of reality, explore the meaning and purpose of your life, and reorganize your priorities and values accordingly. Undoubtedly, this is a demanding, time-consuming task but ultimately an essential one if you are to fully reconcile yourself to the infection and to approach the future honestly and courageously.

Many individuals attempt to reestablish a sense of stability by exploring the real circumstances of how they were infected, of somehow "explaining" their particular situation. Finding a logical sequence of events leading up to the HIV infection confirms that an observable, predictable order does exist. And to a person whose inner vision has suddenly become indistinct and whose belief system has been cast into doubt, this can be very comforting.

Such a search may initially begin in a rather concrete manner. Some people diligently attempt to recall all significant activities and encounters from the past, in an effort to discover when, how, and possibly from whom, they contracted it. You may well find yourself reviewing your own life in detail in this way. When it's not a preoccupation or an attempt to place blame, this type of historical review may actually help you cope with the situation. In addition, it can sometimes yield potentially useful medical information, such as the length of time you may have been infected with the virus. Be wary of becoming obsessed, however; this quest should not interfere with your daily functioning or with other aspects of your life. The inquiry should illuminate, not hinder, and should serve to bring you greater understanding and inner peace.

Having arrived at a satisfactory answer regarding the specific way in which the infection may have occurred, the quest may subsequently turn to the metaphysical realm, with the pursuit of a more profound answer: You may find yourself wondering whether you were *meant* to contract the virus and, if so, why. This concern is not unique to HIV-positive people, but may be found in most anyone who develops a serious illness, who is in a life-threatening situation, or who is confronted with a similar type of personal trauma. The pursuit of spiritual or religious explanations of life's tribulations has commonly been observed in diverse populations and appears to reflect a universal human need to find a cause—a direct and personal reason—when confronted with a painful situation that challenges the integrity of one's view of self and reality and threatens to disrupt the natural flow of life events. For the HIV-positive individual in particular, this inner journey seems to be an essential step toward reconciliation with the infection. Several obstacles exist, however, which may make this process both troubling and difficult.

Because HIV is frequently transmitted through sexual intercourse and the sharing of syringes during drug use, it has become a political magnet for various groups who enhance their identity by denouncing these activities. They cast blame freely on those with HIV, characterizing them as licentious, immoral, and deserving of infection, and undoubtedly this exceedingly harsh and merciless judgment colors the manner in which many infected individuals view themselves. Such pernicious social cruelty can also confuse and disrupt a person's personal search for meaning since it introduces blame, guilt, and divine punishment into an already complex and painful human event.

It is a historical fact that, for several centuries in the Western world, naturally occurring illnesses have frequently been viewed by the masses as displays of religious mystery, "calls to faith," or evidence of God's wrath. Physical illness, then, has been used throughout the ages as a way of bolstering the reigning moral code of a particular society.

Perhaps the most telling example is found in accounts of the bubonic plague—the Black Death—which swept across Europe in the fourteenth century, leaving 24 million deaths in its wake. Today, we know that the plague is caused by a bacteria transmitted to humans through the bite of a flea, and that it is treatable with standard antibiotics. But during the Middle Ages, it was a disease cloaked in mystery and viewed as a judgment from God, a mass punishment for human transgression. In a desperate attempt to purge the evil in the human soul, and hence regain the favor of God, formerly benign individuals felt compelled to engage in barbaric and grotesque acts of violence both on themselves and on others.

In some ways our society is no less harsh in its judgment. HIV infection is generally viewed in a neutral, nonjudgmental manner when it occurs in children and blood transfusion recipients ("innocent victims"); yet it is seen as a form of retribution and punishment when contracted by sexually active adolescents and adults or by intravenous drug users. Obviously, this system of moral interpretation and judgment doesn't make much sense, showing a breakdown in logic that results in a clear double standard. You would therefore be wise to avoid being influenced by such inconsistent, moralistic pronouncements, since they're unproductive and only induce unnecessary guilt that prohibits genuine emotional and spiritual growth.

Sadly, such misguided and judgmental pronouncements cause great harm to real people already struggling with a mortal disease. I saw the kind of turmoil such cruelty causes in Ben, a quiet, gentle young man whose initial emotional reaction to his positive test findings was relatively mild and contained, but who subsequently spent much time attempting to grasp the meaning of his situation intellectually. Like others who harbor the virus, Ben understood how he had contracted it; his question was *why*. In a sense, he felt singled out.

A few weeks after receiving his test results, Ben joined one of our clinic's support groups for gay men. During the first session, he spoke of his confusion and perplexity at having contracted the virus and explained that he sometimes felt as if the infection was a form of punishment. He added, however, that he had reviewed his past and could find nothing in his behavior corrupt enough to warrant such a severe fate.

With the help and support of the other group members, Ben gradually came to throw off this feeling of punishment over the course of a few weeks. He began to view the infection much more rationally, as a medical condition.

Several weeks later, however, Ben abruptly announced

that he had begun yet again to feel as if he were being punished. Furthermore, it appeared that he was becoming increasingly preoccupied with this idea, as he had been prior to entering the group. It had begun to threaten his peace of mind, and he was feeling depressed and having difficulty sleeping.

Inquiring into this sudden, marked regression in his adjustment, I found that these distressing thoughts had apparently been triggered by a televised sermon he had watched, in which a "televangelist" preached a sermon against AIDS. This media figure apparently viewed the illness as a contemporary plague, proclaiming it to be evidence of God's disfavor of homosexuality and drug use, among other practices.

During the group session that followed, the members seemed especially compassionate toward Ben. They adopted a unified stance, informing him that AIDS was not, in their opinion, a divine punishment, and providing logical arguments against the position espoused by the televangelist. They also reminded him that televangelists, like everyone else, are fallible, and cited convincing evidence to support their claim. They emphasized, too, that this view of AIDS as chastisement is not a position uniformly held by all clergy members. Finally, they recommended that, until he had securely reconciled himself with the infection, Ben avoid watching such broadcasts or reading articles that adopt harsh, condemnatory attitudes toward those with HIV infection or AIDS. Throughout this session, these gentlemen warmly offered understanding and love—compassion Ben certainly needed and deserved.

And he did, in fact, follow their advice. At one point, Ben discussed his concerns with a minister he had known for many years, and for whom he felt a great deal of admiration. Later, Ben told me that this discussion had proved to be very reassuring. He continued to attend the support group on a consistent basis, renewing his efforts to understand and reconcile himself to the positive test findings. And lastly, it appeared that, by reducing his exposure to individuals holding negative, caustic views of HIV infection and AIDS, a healing climate emerged in which Ben's mental state and overall adjustment were enhanced.

Even in the absence of overt moral censure from others, however, feelings of punishment or guilt, particularly sexual guilt, sometimes emerge among HIV-infected individuals and can severely impede their progress toward reconciliation. Since HIV can be contracted during sexual intercourse, a powerful connection may be perceived between human sexuality and death, and this association may serve to reactivate many of our sexual traumas and fears dating back to earliest childhood.

When one has had affairs outside of marriage or a committed relationship, for instance, and feels regretful about the deception, the infection may be experienced as a punishment. In much the same way, a person who has not fully accepted his or her homosexual feelings may experience the infection as a form of retribution for that form of sexual contact. Since our society often encourages shame and self-reproach in sexually active individuals, especially those having alternative sexual preferences, feelings of guilt and self-loathing have already been instilled in many of us. To contract a sexually transmitted infection, then, may serve to confirm one's sense of deviance and worthlessness, and thus further undermine an individual's self-esteem and overall adjustment.

While "healthy" guilt does exist and is a characteristic of mature moral development, most guilt is of the unhealthy or neurotic kind. By its nature, neurotic guilt markedly inhibits emotional development and its associated feelings of shame and self-reproach can prevent you from progressing emotionally or spiritually. If this description sounds like the circumstances you're presently caught up in, you would probably benefit from some type of counseling. Effective professional intervention may help alleviate the unnecessary self-blame and free you to proceed with your quest for meaning.

A second potential obstacle concerns the current "commercialization" of AIDS as it interferes with each person's individualized search for understanding. Because there are now millions of HIV-infected individuals worldwide and millions more lovers, relatives, and friends of those infected, a sizable consumer market exists. It is now common for lectures, videotapes, cassette tapes, and written publications to attempt to provide global emotional or spiritual answers for HIV-positive persons, with the proposed solutions invariably designed to reestablish a sense of individual power, control, and self-determination. In my experience, however, the only answers that ultimately hold any truth or endure are those that come from meaningful personal experience and inner contemplation. Only from questioning, searching, analyzing, and deliberating, will you arrive at genuine truths.

Rather than deferring to the opinions of others, you should approach the search independently. While this certainly does not imply that you should isolate yourself from the views of others, it does suggest that you must finally arrive at an understanding of your situation based on your own deliberations. Of course, you may wish to seek counsel and guidance from other HIV-positive persons or from a therapist, priest, rabbi, or other clergy member; indeed, this may prove immensely helpful. Most important, though, is that the understanding you ultimately reap, whenever it may be, bring with it feelings of vibrancy, clarity, and truth.

Obviously, as individuals with HIV discover their own meanings for the condition, what seems valid to one person may be altogether untenable to another. This is irrelevant, however, since the goal of the adjustment process is to achieve a reconciliation with one's own HIV condition. To generalize your insights to all others infected with HIV, though probably well-intentioned, is nevertheless to disregard the importance of the unique journeys of your peers. It may even hinder their development. Likewise, to adopt another person's viewpoint without reaching it through your own contemplation is to assume a perspective that may be contrary to your innermost feelings and beliefs.

In my experience, individuals infected with HIV arrive at a wide spectrum of answers to the question, "Why me?" For a few, the infection is, at least briefly, interpreted as a punishment, while for others it comes to be viewed as a harbinger of a new and unique purpose to their lives. For one it may be an opportunity to explore certain aspects or dimensions of existence, while for another it may be seen as an act of providence through which he or she is influenced to pursue a specific course of action. Of course, to many there appears to be no underlying metaphysical meaning whatsoever, with the virus being viewed simply as an infectious agent, and their infection as due to the "odds" or chance. Aside from these differences in perspective, however, most people do arrive at an understanding or resolution of some kind, which helps them accept and live with the infection. In most instances, it assists in restoring a sense of security and stability to their lives, while also orienting them toward the future. Your own answers, it is hoped, will assist you in living fully and productively with the HIV condition as well.

Renewal

Once you have made peace with the positive test findings as part of your life, and once the emotional turmoil has dissipated, you will probably begin to feel reconciled with the infection. This does not mean that you embrace the condition or are in resounding harmony with it, but rather that you have resigned yourself to it and both recognize and respect its reality. At this point, you will have become able to continue your life with greater security and inner peace.

To some infected individuals the possibility of eventual illness now seems a distant abstraction and is no longer a major issue. For others, however, awareness of the infection remains uppermost in their mind, with the specter of developing an HIV-related illness looming in the shadows. Ironically, such a keen awareness of one's HIV condition often has the indirect effect of enhancing a person's existence. Sharply attuned to the reality of future illness, an individual may come to place much more value and immediacy on life itself. No longer taking other people or events for granted, the person may enter the bittersweet position of embracing and loving life far more deeply and sincerely, simply because of the realization that we are all mortal.

While being infected is certainly not a desirable condition, it does provide you with an opportunity usually unavailable to those who are not infected with HIV: to be able, while still in fine health, to glimpse the prospect of mortality and to appreciate and live your life more richly, completely, and intensely as a result. You may form genuinely meaningful relationships with others, realizing that the bonds may not last forever, and therefore nurturing and cherishing the relationships and their moments more deeply than you might have prior to this experience.

You may also find yourself wishing to mend damaged relationships from the past. Some infected individuals reconcile old grievances with parents and siblings, forgiving long-ago mistakes or hurts so as to restore loving, life-affirming relationships with their families. Others wish to heal broken relationships with ex-spouses, lovers, or friends. Some infected persons are even able to forgive themselves of their own faults and shortcomings and in the process they become once again able to accept themselves.

This blossoming out can also be seen in an HIV-positive person's change to become more assertive, as well as politically or humanistically involved in various activities. In most cases, the individual also adopts an activist stance aimed at preserving his or her mental and physical well-being in an effort to counter the progression of the infection itself. Such an attitude is psychologically healthy and may well serve to enhance the quality of one's life and to extend it.

In essence, the goal is to live each moment fully and completely, to seek out and make use of those medical treatments available, and to practice a way of life that enhances physical and mental health. Thousands of HIV-positive persons choose to approach their lives in this manner, electing to embrace and build on the knowledge of their conditions and maintaining their state of good health until a cure, or at least other significant treatment, becomes available to arrest the infection.

The Judeo-Christian tradition tells the story of Job, a man laden with overwhelming obstacles and unrelenting responsibilities. Unable to understand why he was being so burdened, Job believed that he was being punished by God and thus spent much time searching for the reasons behind his apparent chastisement. In actuality, Job's suffering was a gift, since it was through this painful struggle that he became closer to his inner self and to the ultimate nature of his God.

Interpreting the Book of Job, Jungian psychoanalyst Edward Edinger, M.D., says that the Scriptures were "a record of a divine initiation process, a testing by ordeal, which when successful leads to a new state of being. . . . The favorites of God receive the severest ordeals." Dr. Edinger adds that "Job asked why his misery should happen to him. The answer that emerges from the Book of Job is so that he may see God [1]."

Rabbi Harold Kushner offers another view of personal misfortune, a view that illuminates its effects. "Pain is the price we pay for being alive," he writes. "We may not ever understand why we suffer or be able to control the forces that cause our suffering, but we can have a lot to say about what the suffering does to us, and what sort of people we become because of it [2]."

Through the challenge of HIV-positivity, you may come to know yourself, your loved ones, and the essence of life itself. Paradoxically, your fear and doubt may well give rise to renewed strength, direction, and purpose. Confronting and prevailing over this momentous obstacle may require a great deal of you, but by maintaining faith in yourself and in your convictions, you may deepen and expand tremendously, emerging more fulfilled, more aware, and more fully alive than at any time in your life.

7

When a Loved One Tests Positive for HIV

When a person with whom you share a personal relationship undergoes testing for HIV infection, the experience may be stressful not only for your loved one but for you as well. Whether it be a friend, relative, lover, or spouse, the complex emotional journey on which they are embarking will most likely have an impact on you, quite possibly a profound and enduring one. In a similar manner, your own response to the situation may influence your loved one's adjustment powerfully. If you hold back emotions or express your own anger and fear in harsh feelings inadvertently directed at them, you may undermine their ability to cope with the situation. Your genuine expressions of love, concern, and acceptance on the other hand, lend strength and a sense of protection and shelter during this stormy period.

As a rule, it appears that most people find it easier

to respond with understanding and nurturance to a friend or family member who undergoes HIV testing than to a lover or spouse, since presumably one is not sexually involved with the former. When you have been sexually active with a person being tested, or have shared other potential routes of infection, the situation may become much more complicated. In fact, it can be emotionally intense, since you both may experience similar psychological reactions to the person's assessment process. For this reason, we will distinguish between nonsexual and sexual relationships in our discussion of emotional support.

Nonsexual Relationships

When people decide to be tested, it is not unusual for them to keep this information to themselves. This is not necessarily from a lack of trust but instead may show that they are not yet emotionally prepared to approach the topic with others or simply don't want to worry friends or relatives. Conversely, when a loved one does, in fact, reveal his or her assessment plans to you, you should consider the likely possibility that the person is apprehensive and indirectly requesting your support and assistance.

AWAITING THE TEST RESULTS

Before the test, the person may display any of several emotions, ranging from a seeming lack of concern to outright panic. Such emotional expressions may persist, even increase, during the days or weeks before the results come back. An especially lengthy interval between testing and results may escalate an individual's anxiety even further.

During this period, your loved one may become preoccupied with the HIV test and may temporarily withdraw from others and want to be alone. Don't interpret this withdrawal, which may be both abrupt and total, as a personal rejection or as necessarily undesirable or unhealthy but rather as their simple need for solitude during a crucial period. Creating a quiet space free of outside responsibilities and concerns affords the individual an opportunity to reflect on the current situation, to weigh the possible meanings and implications of the impending test findings, and to prepare to accept the findings as part of his or her life. Thus, it marks the beginning of the adjustment process and forms the foundation for coping with those additional stresses that may emerge as events unfold. For many, there is a conscious decision to undertake this early psychological preparation alone or with only limited help from others. You should respect this choice and, as a dedicated friend or relative, take your cues from your loved one. You should strive to be available when he or she solicits your attention and support, while allowing the person uninterrupted privacy, detachment, and distance when this is asked or implied.

More rarely, a person will prefer to be around others when feeling apprehensive about the upcoming results and will throw themselves into social or career activities in a conspicuously frenetic manner. As a method of obtaining emotional comfort and an escape from recurrent thoughts or worries about the HIV test, this may be the only way they feel able to contend with the stress of testing. Again, you can best help by creating an atmosphere of understanding and acceptance, by providing affection and a sense of security, and by reassuring the person of your continued presence during and after the assessment process.

On some occasions, you may notice that the person is more irritable, argumentative, or angry than usual; these are expressions of the marked tension associated with the assessment. During such times, be patient and yielding, and this may be remarkably effective in defusing much of this hostility and easing the emotional strain your friend or relative is enduring. Without assuming a patronizing stance, it is important that you be both tolerant and forgiving in your encounters with your loved one, even though this may be difficult at times. Ultimately, your aim should be to help the person avoid stress as much as possible, so that his or her energies might be directed exclusively toward coping with issues related to the testing. Avoiding arguments, eliminating unnecessary emotional or social demands, and refraining from excessive advice-giving or lecturing may greatly aid in this effort.

WHEN THE RESULTS ARE NEGATIVE

When the test findings come in, you can expect your loved one to show a visible emotional release if the test is negative, most commonly a reaction of overwhelming relief, even jubilation. Some people will then vow to ensure their continued good health by modifying their life-styles—eating well, exercising, stopping bad habits, practicing safer sex. You may notice any of these life-affirming changes in your loved one, too, and you would be performing a truly beneficial deed if you were to support these resolutions.

WHEN THE RESULTS ARE POSITIVE

In contrast, the person receiving positive test findings may well be temporarily emotionally devastated. Since the diversity of such reactions has been discussed at length in Chapter 6, it is not necessary to reiterate them here. Suffice it to say, the most frequent responses include fear, confusion, hopelessness, and despair.

As a concerned friend or family member, you must understand the gravity of your loved one's situation. For that person, contending with a positive test can be demanding and laborious, since it is no less than a confrontation with mortality, a part of reality for which few of us are prepared. For many of us, our entire lives may be spent avoiding such realizations, but for the individual who tests HIV-positive, fundamental existential issues often come to the fore, presenting an intense emotional and spiritual challenge. It is impossible, of course, for you to share fully your loved one's inner experience; instead, you must remain in the role of a concerned outsider, being available for your loved one to lean on and providing emotional sustenance as much as you can. Still, your presence itself may be deeply reassuring, since it reaffirms the bond you share and anchors the person in the immediate reality of the relationship.

For you, the experience may also be stressful, confusing, and disheartening. Sadly enough, it does happen that friends and family of those who test HIV-positive avoid their loved ones, either from a groundless fear of contracting the infection or, more often, from a sense of perplexity about how to behave around them. In some cases, a relative or friend may be quite upset and saddened by a loved one's positive test findings, in which case it is best to temporarily stay away from the person in order to avoid adding to their emotional burden. This is the exception, however, and you should try, as best you can, to put your own feelings aside for the moment to offer full support to your friend or relative. This is because, regardless of the reason one avoids an individual who tests positive, the infected person invariably feels shunned or rejected—at the precise moment when human contact may be needed most desperately.

If you are overwhelmed by your loved one's test findings and aren't sure how to act, remember that simply being with the person and listening to their concerns can be immensely helpful. You can also be instructive, recognizing and correcting any misconceptions they may hold about the meaning and implications of the test findings. Remind the person that testing HIV-positive is not synonymous with a diagnosis of AIDS; that the two conditions are distinct. Since your loved one may be emotionally distraught and somewhat irrational, you should try to stay calm and be a reassuring presence, lending your sense of reason to the situation.

There are other concerns as well. Even though you will need to express your own thoughts and fears upon hearing the news that a loved one has tested positive, you must consider very seriously that they may have chosen you, and only you, to tell. You must respect their wishes by not revealing the test findings to anyone else, under any circumstances. If you need to discuss your own feelings with someone else, then you should do so in a way that preserves your loved one's privacy.

In essence, this time may be quite taxing for both of you. But it is a time when you can truly help another person, a very special one in this case. For it is through your relationship that you may help heal an emotionally and spiritually wounded person; it is a truly generous and noble act, a gift of love. And as a result, you may find your relationship deepening and strengthening; the bond between you and your loved one can grow, expand, and transcend what came before.

Sexual Relationships

When you are involved in a sexual relationship with someone who receives positive test findings you may find the situation extremely distressing, since your own HIV status also comes into question. Consequently, it may be difficult, if not impossible, for you to remain composed, patient, and empathic. You may instead feel restless and worried, with relatively limited emotional resources to offer your intimate.

If the two of you have engaged in any of the sexual practices that transmit the infection, you should strongly consider being tested. If your test findings are negative, you will be in a more secure position to provide assistance and emotional support. If your test findings are positive, however, you may both wish to seek counseling, since it may be very hard for you to sustain each other when stressed by such circumstances.

WHEN YOUR PARTNER TESTS HIV-POSITIVE

If your partner tests positive, you may cope with the situation in either a maladaptive or an adaptive manner, depending on a variety of factors. Especially if your own test results prove to be negative, you may find yourself inwardly reviewing your relationship with your HIV-positive partner and possibly considering terminating it. Sometimes people panic when they realize that the person with whom they live and make love is infected with HIV, and some impulsively and abruptly abandon the relationship. This is an irrational act based on fear, and it is also exceedingly cruel as well as unnecessary, since the relationship may well have flourished despite the adversity. If you do feel an urgent need to flee from your relationship, try at least temporarily to control the impulse and attempt to conquer your anxieties. A decision of such mutual importance should be reached only after careful deliberation and discussion with your partner. And should you eventually decide to leave, you should do it as gently as possible, minimizing its deleterious effects on your partner.

Of course, you may well decide to remain in the relationship, as many do. And if you choose to stay, you must take measures to prevent your own infection, with sexual practices usually requiring the most substantial modification. As a couple, you may decide to abstain from sexual relations completely or to engage in risk-free sex only. You should examine nonsexual areas of your life together to determine if there are other ways that you might be exposed to your partner's infection, and eliminate these risks. Discussing your lifestyle with an HIV counselor could help you identify and modify any such potentially hazardous activities.

As you and your partner adapt to the situation creatively and flexibly, together you may gradually incorporate the positive test findings into the fabric of your relationship. It is reassuring to note that thousands of couples are currently living harmoniously with one partner infected with HIV and the other partner free from infection.

WHEN BOTH YOU AND YOUR PARTNER TEST HIV-POSITIVE

When you and your partner both test positive, the strain on your relationship can be truly burdensome.

Depending on how the two of you address the test results, your relationship may weaken under the stress and suffer mightily, or it may weather the troubling event and become newly energized and vital.

Particularly if you both receive your test findings at about the same time, the relationship may well enter an acute period of crisis. The situation will be even more bleak if you interpret the positive test findings in the worst possible light—as meaning impending illness or death. At this time, you or your partner may need some emotional distance from the relationship, at least temporarily.

In some instances, one or both partners, perhaps wishing to evade the harsh reality of the test findings, will feel a need to break the ties. Sometimes the unendurable stress of living with a partner who is infected with HIV—being reminded of one's own condition on virtually a daily basis—leads to the breakup. Avoiding the partner may seem to provide a means of escaping the unpleasant fact of the positive test results but at the same time it cuts off a principal source of support at precisely the moment when it might be most valuable. Of course, such avoidance also stops you from facing up to the positive findings and coming to terms with them. Rejecting your partner might leave you in the end with no option but to confront the test findings alone, without the comfort and guidance provided by a mutually supportive, intimate relationship.

A second problem that you may find in your relationship pertains to the source of the infection. Occasionally, one person blames the other for the infection, and the relationship founders because of the hostility that ensues. If you know that sexual infidelity is what resulted in HIV infection, for instance, then your sense of trust and commitment may be critically undermined and the partnership jeopardized. Indeed, it may not be salvageable.

The case of Gerard and Anne-Marie illustrates this process. The couple had been married for four years when Anne-Marie learned that her husband was involved with another woman. Their marriage was threatened by this discovery, of course, but was prevented from collapsing when Gerard renounced the affair and reaffirmed his commitment to the marriage.

Then, nearly eleven years later, while attempting to donate blood, he learned that he was infected with HIV. Gerard explained the situation to Anne-Marie, who became extremely anxious and upset. She quickly scheduled an appointment for herself at our HIV testing agency.

Fortunately, Anne-Marie's test findings were negative, and she was clearly relieved. Nevertheless, she told me that she still had several serious concerns; among them, when and how her husband had become infected and whether he had been involved in other sexual liaisons besides the one earlier in their marriage.

Several months later, Anne-Marie returned to our agency to be retested for HIV infection, to confirm the findings from the original assessment. The results were again negative.

During this second visit, Anne-Marie discussed the state of her marriage since Gerard's positive test. At her request, she and Gerard were now living apart but were meeting weekly with a marital therapist. Further, Anne-Marie had not yet decided if she wished to return to the marriage. Gerard, she said, had admitted to a history of fleeting extramarital relationships, and she found this unacceptable. She added that, although she could handle Gerard's infection, she couldn't handle living in a marriage with a husband she didn't trust. Consequently, trust, rather than HIV infection, emerged as the core issue for her.

Even when infidelity is not a factor, there may still be a tendency for one or both partners to assign blame out of fear, frustration, and anger at being infected. Using the partner as a target for reproach, however, is unkind, unfair, and deeply destructive, and may well make the partner's adjustment far more arduous. It may also induce a sense of guilt in the person, worsening any feelings of depression and dejection.

You and your loved one should try to accept the test results without ascribing blame or avoiding each other. By relying on each other for assistance, encouragement, and emotional sustenance, your relationship may not only survive this event relatively intact but may even become increasingly durable with time. Thus, by contending with the test findings with maturity, compassion, and a sense of shared responsibility, you are much more likely to prosper together in a secure future relationship—one that possesses an inherent resiliency and is better able to withstand those medical or other stresses that may come.

When the two of you receive positive HIV test results, it is also a timely occasion to initiate life-style changes directed at controlling and containing the infection. For instance, a productive relationship in which both partners are infected with HIV is usually characterized by a sexual life restricted to activities that will not reinfect the partners; they engage in low-risk or risk-free sexual behaviors to avoid passing more of the virus to one another during sexual relations because it is believed by some scientists that repeated contact with

HIV increases the amount of virus in the bloodstream, thus increasing the likelihood of illness. They also tend to encourage other behavioral changes in each other to maintain and enhance their overall health and well-being. Such modifications may mean eating healthier foods, getting exercise, learning stress management, and related activities too. And finally, a heterosexual couple may decide to have their children tested, if there exists the possibility that their children were exposed to HIV during pregnancy or childbirth. Realistic measures of this kind show that a couple is confronting the infection and adopting measures to inhibit its effects and prevent its spread.

Together, you may decide to make similar adaptive life-style changes in your own relationship. You might also consider seeking brief supportive or problem-solving therapy from a mental health professional or a counselor at an HIV/AIDS testing and counseling center to accelerate, and possibly enhance, your adjustment to the situation. An alternative is a support group for HIV-positive individuals or couples, an avenue that could prove especially valuable. Above all, though, you must allow your intimate relationship the time and freedom to adjust to the test findings in much the same way that you, as an individual, will need a certain period of time to accept and live with the information.

The Essence of Human Love

While there exists a spectrum of pleasant emotions we rather airily refer to as "love," in fact, genuine human love—that which one person feels deeply and intensely for another person—is quite exceptional, tending to be reserved for the most treasured people who pass through one's life. And it is such love that ultimately binds us to one another.

Regardless of gender, race, age, or sexual preference, we all share a fundamental human need to give and to receive affection and to establish a sense of security in our intimate relationships. By our natures and by our circumstances, we are all ultimately dependent on one another for sustenance and strength. During times of hardship and misfortune this interdependency becomes manifest, and the need for human contact becomes most urgent. Solidarity thus becomes paramount to ensure that we survive and surmount events that threaten to shatter our lives.

Your HIV-positive friend, relative, lover, or spouse needs you, and you are most likely in a good position to provide immense help to this special person. Indeed, it is your human responsibility to intervene. Love is not merely an emotion; it is a call to action, an altruistic obligation to provide for the growth and the fulfillment of another. And at a time when those infected with HIV or suffering from AIDS tend to be the victims of social and political intolerance it is particularly important that you meet such pervasive destructiveness with acts of affirmation, generosity, and goodwill.

During those cold, black nights of the soul, when one is most truly alone, a piercing awareness of one's isolation in the world may suddenly burst into consciousness and reverberate through one's being. Yet through the grace of human contact, such a chilling insight may be quelled, at least momentarily, and warmth and light returned to the soul. To afford such solace to a frightened, struggling person is to perform an act of extraordinary human kindness; to accept such comfort is to receive mercy and strength; and to share such a bond is to experience the essence of human love.

8

Questions and Answers About HIV Testing

Questions that commonly arise in discussions of HIV testing are presented in this chapter, and brief answers are provided. You can refer to the preceding text for a fuller explanation.

What Is HIV?

HIV stands for Human Immunodeficiency Virus, the virus that causes AIDS. There are two principal types of this virus: HIV-1, which is prevalent in North America and Europe; and HIV-2, which is widespread in certain parts of Africa. Both are formidable agents and may cause irreparable damage to a person's immune system.

How Does One Contract HIV?

HIV is most often contracted through direct, intimate contact with an infected person's blood, semen, or vagi-

114

nal fluids. Penetrative sexual acts, intravenous drug use, and pregnancy and childbirth are among the most common means of viral transmission. Prior to 1985, contaminated blood products, including blood transfusions, were also a significant cause of HIV infection.

How Long Does HIV Infection Last?

It is believed that, once infected with the human immunodeficiency virus, a person remains infected for life. Researchers currently have evidence that the individual continues to be infectious to others throughout his or her lifetime.

What Is the Difference Between HIV Infection and AIDS?

HIV infection simply means that the virus is present in a person's bloodstream. Most HIV-infected people, despite the fact that they harbor the virus in their bodies, are otherwise healthy and do not have symptoms of AIDS.

Several years after becoming infected, people sometimes find that the long-term presence of the virus has gradually eroded their immune systems. They become increasingly unable to combat infection and are vulnerable to a variety of maladies. At this point, AIDS-related complex (ARC) or AIDS may become the diagnosis. Symptoms of illness must always be present before AIDS can be diagnosed.

Why Is HIV Infection Associated with Homosexuality?

One of the earliest North American subpopulations to be affected by the virus was that of gay men in major urban centers. Since that time, we have come to realize that heterosexual men and women, as well as children, are just as vulnerable to the virus; HIV infection is not limited to any particular sexual preference. Still, the misleading association between HIV and homosexuality persists in some quarters and will, we hope, be corrected through continued public health education.

How Do I Know if I Have Been Infected with HIV?

It is common for an infected person to carry the virus for several years without experiencing noticeable symptoms. In fact, an extremely large number of people are presumed to be infected but unaware of it because of a lack of symptoms. Consequently, the only way to know with certainty whether you are infected is to have an HIV test.

What Is an HIV Test?

An HIV test is a technique that reveals whether a person is infected with the human immunodeficiency virus by analyzing particular body fluids, such as blood. At the present time, there are several types of HIV tests. Some detect actual components of the virus itself, while others measure the body's response to the virus (e.g., EIA or ELISA, Western blot technique). These latter measures, called "antibody tests," are most common, because they are easy to perform and economical to use. The findings from antibody tests are classified as "positive," "negative," or "inconclusive" ("indeterminate").

What Is the "AIDS Test"?

There is no AIDS test. AIDS is diagnosed when a person displays specific physical symptoms, in conjunction with the presence of identifiable risk factors, blood test results, and findings from additional laboratory studies.

The term "AIDS Test" is actually a misnomer and incorrectly refers to tests for HIV infection. And HIV infection is distinct from AIDS.

Can an HIV Test Predict if I Will Develop AIDS?

An HIV test can reveal if you are infected with the human immunodeficiency virus. It cannot determine how long you have been infected nor if or when you will develop symptoms of AIDS.

What Does a Positive Test Result Mean?

A positive test finding indicates that the virus has, at some previous time, entered one's bloodstream. Presumably, it is still present in the body and will remain so indefinitely. A person who receives a positive test result is considered to be HIV-infected.

Less often, a positive test finding is the result of a technical error in the laboratory that processes the blood test or of the interaction of certain other medical problems or unusual properties in the blood itself with the test to produce a false-positive finding. For this reason confirmatory tests should always be performed.

What Should I Do if I Test HIV-Positive?

If you test positive, you should work closely with your HIV counselor or physician to plan a specific course of action. Arrangements often include a medical examination performed by a doctor familiar with HIV. The evaluation normally includes a TB skin test and a T-cell count (a procedure used to determine the current status of the immune system). In some cases, medication to slow the infection may be prescribed. Finally, you should change your life-style to bolster the immune system and otherwise enhance your health.

What Are the Medical Treatments for HIV Infection?

There are currently several treatments available for those infected with HIV. Among the most effective are drugs that slow the virus from reproducing within the body, thereby delaying the deleterious effects of the infection for months or years.

If I Test Positive for HIV and Need Help Coping with It, Where Can I Find Assistance?

An HIV counselor or an AIDS hotline can provide you with information concerning the available support resources in your local area. Many community HIV/AIDS testing and counseling agencies offer individual counseling or support groups for those infected with the virus, with such help being very effective in many cases. Depending on your situation, you might also wish to seek the support of someone in your family or circle of friends, if you would feel comfortable disclosing your test results to these people. Finally, private therapists can always provide beneficial psychological services during stressful times.

What Does a Negative Test Result Mean?

In most cases, a negative antibody test result indicates that a person is not infected with HIV. There are instances, however, when a test may produce a false-negative result although the person is actually infected. This may occur when a person is tested too early in the course of the infection, or when certain other medical problems interfere with the test. Occasionally, an individual in the advanced stages of AIDS obtains a negative antibody test result due to the depletion of antibody in the bloodstream.

It is important to note that a negative finding does not mean that one is immune to the virus.

If a Negative Finding May Be Wrong, Why Should I Be Tested At All?

In most cases, a negative finding is accurate—the person is not infected with HIV. In those instances when the negative result is questionable, however, periodic retesting will almost always clarify one's true HIV status.

Furthermore, since there is always the possibility, whenever a person is tested, that a positive test finding may be obtained, this alone makes testing worthwhile; a positive finding signals the presence of infection and the need for medical attention.

What Does an Inconclusive or Indeterminate Test Result Mean?

An inconclusive or indeterminate test result means that an antibody test cannot determine whether infection is present in the blood sample. Accidents or errors in the laboratory, certain other illnesses or unusual characteristics of the blood unrelated to HIV infection, or an insufficient amount of antibody in the blood sample are a few of the causes of inconclusive or indeterminate test findings. Typically, a person is requested to repeat the test or is urged to undergo other types of assessment in order to determine conclusively his or her HIV status. An individual who is not at high risk for infection and who continues to receive indeterminate findings for six months or longer is usually considered to be uninfected.

What Is the Primary Advantage of Being Tested for HIV Infection?

The principal advantage of HIV testing is that it tells

you whether or not you are infected with the human immunodeficiency virus, thereby indicating the need for life-style modification and, possibly, early medical intervention. In much the same way, a negative test result may serve as a significant impetus for change. Regardless of the nature of the test finding, then, the results of an HIV test often play a decisive role in redirecting a person's life.

Should I Be Tested for HIV Infection?

You should consider being tested for infection if you have reason to believe that you may have been in contact with the virus and if you further believe that you would be able to cope with a positive test result. If you feel uncertain about whether you have been in close contact with HIV or if you have doubts about your ability to contend with the test finding, it is recommended that you call an AIDS hotline or arrange a meeting with an HIV counselor or physician to discuss your questions and concerns.

Those commonly advised to seek testing include the following: Anyone who has engaged in unsafe sexual behavior in recent years, intravenous drugs users, persons having histories of sexually transmitted diseases, couples planning marriage or pregnancy, those in the sex industry, and prison inmates. Also, hemophiliacs and others who received blood, blood products, or tissue transplants between 1978 and 1985 may be at risk and in need of testing.

It should be noted that the tests commonly used in the United States and Europe measure infection with HIV-1. The other major strain of the virus, HIV-2, is rare in the United States but is prevalent in parts of western Africa. Consequently, if you have had potentially infectious contact with a person from western Africa, then you might consider being tested for HIV-2 in addition to HIV-1. Today, antibody tests exist that are designed to measure both types.

How Long Should I Wait Before Taking an HIV Test?

Once HIV enters the body, it may reach a testable level in two weeks, but normally a person is advised to wait four to twelve weeks before being tested. The reason is to allow the body adequate time to develop antibody and thus increase the likelihood of an accurate test result.

You should be aware that in some cases, up to six months have elapsed before an individual's body has produced a measurable level of antibody. For this reason, you may consider being retested approximately six months after the date of your last possible contact with the virus.

What Does Undergoing an HIV Test Entail?

A standard HIV antibody test is simple and brief, since the test requires only a blood sample. Furthermore, testing to confirm a positive finding is typically performed using the same blood sample.

How Much Does It Cost to Take an HIV Test?

The cost of HIV testing varies greatly, depending on the setting in which it is conducted. At a community HIV/AIDS testing center, an assessment may be free of charge or may involve a nominal fee or donation. Being tested by a physician or a private medical facility, in contrast, may be costlier. Currently, fees range from under $5.00 at certain government-funded facilities up to $200.00 at private medical facilities. Call in advance to determine the costs at the site you choose.

Can I Be Required to Take an HIV Test?

Testing for HIV Infection is mandatory under certain circumstances, such as application to the U.S. military; in some cases, during physical examinations for individual health or life insurance; or certain types of employment. Occasionally, people choose to undergo HIV testing voluntarily and anonymously at an independent agency prior to submitting to mandatory testing to learn the test results in advance. If the results prove to be positive, they can cancel the mandatory testing session, thereby protecting their privacy.

You should be aware that certain insurance companies, when determining if an individual is a candidate for an individual health or life insurance policy, may decide to limit or deny coverage to an individual infected with the human immunodeficiency virus.

Why Is Privacy Such an Important Issue in HIV Testing?

Since the beginning of the North American and European AIDS epidemics, unprecedented discrimination has confronted those with HIV infection and AIDS. In recent years, some individuals testing HIV-positive have been treated with blatant inhumanity, injustice, and contempt by their communities. Therefore, if you're considering undergoing an HIV test, you should consider keeping this decision to yourself.

Furthermore, when an individual receives a positive result on an HIV test, signifying infection, the person should be especially circumspect when revealing this to others. People have lost their insurance, jobs, and housing because of positive test findings. Until our society adopts a more mature, humane, and realistic view of HIV infection, and until our government is willing to provide sufficient legal protection for those who are infected, you should be cautious telling anyone you don't know or trust.

What Is The Difference Between Anonymous Testing and Confidential Testing?

Some HIV test sites offer anonymity while others offer confidentiality. Of the two, anonymity is preferable.

In anonymous testing, the name of the individual being tested is never known. Instead, a code number or other form of nontraceable identification is assigned, and this identification is used throughout the assessment process.

In contrast, the name of the individual is known to the test agency using confidentiality. However, the person's identity and test results are usually protected from disclosure to outside sources unless the test recipient specifically authorizes the release of this information.

Where Can I Undergo an HIV Test?

In many cities and towns, testing for HIV infection is offered at agencies specifically designed for this purpose. Such HIV/AIDS testing and counseling centers typically offer complete assessment services, including individual counseling before and after the test, at little or no cost to the client. Many private physicians' offices also perform HIV tests, as do public health clinics. And finally, HIV tests are sometimes offered in drug-dependence and sexually-transmitted disease clinics, tuberculosis centers, hospitals, and family planning agencies.

123

Blood Banks Routinely Test All Donors for HIV Infection, Can I Donate Blood to Find Out if I Am Infected?

Under no circumstances should you donate blood to learn if you are HIV-infected. Donating blood that may contain the human immunodeficiency virus is a potentially dangerous act and is considered a felony in some states. If you wish to know if you are infected with the virus, then you should seek testing at an agency designed to provide such services, or should consult your doctor or other medical resource.

What Should I Require of an HIV Testing Site?

When selecting a test site, you should choose an agency that strictly adheres to anonymous, or at least confidential, testing procedures. You should also choose one that provides individual counseling before and after the test, so that you will understand the nature of HIV infection and antibody testing and will have emotional support available to you throughout the assessment process. As part of its policy, the agency should also routinely retest all HIV-positive test findings to confirm their accuracy. Finally, the site should be capable of providing psychological, social, and medical services to those who test HIV positive or should be in a position to refer the individual to such resources.

Appendix A

Available Resources

National AIDS Information Hotline
English: (800) 342-AIDS
Spanish: (800) 344-SIDA
Hearing-Impaired: (800) 243-7889

American Civil Liberties Union (ACLU):
AIDS Project
132 West 43rd Street
New York, New York 10036
(212) 944-9800

Lambda Legal Defense and Education Fund
666 Broadway, 12th Floor
New York, New York 10012
(212) 995-8585

Military Law Task Force:
National Military Task Force on AIDS
1168 Union Street, Suite 201
San Diego, California 92101
(619) 233-1701

Appendix A

National Gay and Lesbian Task Force
1734 14th Street N.W.
Washington, D.C. 20009
(202) 332-6483

National Hemophilia Foundation
110 Greene Street, Room 406
New York, New York 10012
(212) 219-8180

National Task Force on Prostitution/Coyote
333 Valencia Street, Suite 101
San Francisco, California 94103
(415) 558-0450

Appendix B

HIV Test Reporting Practices, by State (U.S.A.)*

GROUP 1:
States that require the names of HIV-positive individuals to be reported to the local or state health department

Alabama	Minnesota	South Carolina
Arizona	Mississippi	South Dakota
Arkansas	Missouri	Utah
Colorado	North Carolina	Virginia
Idaho	North Dakota	West Virginia
Indiana	Ohio	Wisconsin
Michigan	Oklahoma	Wyoming

---

*Information obtained from the Centers of Disease Control (*Morbidity and Mortality Weekly Report,* vol. 39, no. 47, p. 859). This material represents reporting laws as of 1 October 1990.

GROUP 2:

States that do not require the names of HIV-positive persons to be reported, but do require other, non-personal information to be provided (demographic and transmission data)

Georgia	Kentucky	New Jersey
Illinois	Maine	Oregon
Iowa	Montana	Rhode Island
Kansas	Nevada	Texas

GROUP 3:

States that do not require names or HIV test results to be reported to local or state health departments

Alaska	Hawaii	New Mexico
California	Louisiana	New York
Connecticut	Maryland	Pennsylvania
Delaware	Massachusetts	Tennessee
District of Columbia	Nebraska	Vermont
Florida	New Hampshire	Washington

NOTE: New Jersey has passed a law mandating the reporting of positive HIV test results by name, but the law has not yet been implemented. Also, Maryland and Washington require the names of HIV-positive persons who have actual symptoms of illness to be reported.

Because reporting laws do change, it is advisable that you contact your local or state health department before being tested, to determine its current laws.

Glossary

AIDS: Acquired Immune Deficiency Syndrome.

ANTIBODY: A protein produced by the immune system, which fights infection by combining with and incapacitating the agents that cause infection.

ARC: AIDS-Related Complex. The term is being used less than previously; ARC refers to symptoms of HIV infection that are not so serious or pronounced as to suggest a diagnosis of AIDS. Symptoms of ARC often include fever, enlarged lymph nodes, diarrhea, and weight loss.

CARRIER: An otherwise healthy person who harbors an infection and who is capable of spreading the infection to others.

CONTAGION: The spread of infection through direct contact.

EPIDEMIC: A very large number of cases of a particular disease within a specified geographic region.

EPIDEMIOLOGY: The study of the various factors that contribute to the occurrence and spread of disease within the population.

HEMOPHILIA: A hereditary disorder characterized by an inability of the blood to coagulate, or clot, properly. Most often, this disorder is found in males.

HIV: The Human Immunodeficiency Virus, the agent that causes AIDS. Two strains of the virus have been identified: HIV-1, which is prevalent in North America and Europe; and HIV-2, which is common in parts of western Africa.

HOST: A species that is capable of being infected by a particular agent.

IMMUNE SYSTEM: The system within the human body that preserves health by fighting disease. One means by which the immune system resists illness is through the creation of antibody to attack specific viruses that threaten one's health.

IMMUNITY: The ability to resist disease.

IMMUNODEFICIENCY: A state of impairment or dysfunction of the immune system.

INCIDENCE: The number of cases of a disease occurring within a given time frame.

INFECTION: The process whereby a foreign agent lodges and reproduces within a host.

INFECTIVITY: The ability of a foreign agent, such as a virus, to infect a host.

INTRAMUSCULAR: Into the muscle.

INTRAVENOUS: Into the vein.

PANDEMIC: A large-scale epidemic, usually of global proportions.

PORTAL OF ENTRY: The means by which a foreign agent, such as a virus, enters a host.

SCREENING TEST: A method for the rapid identification of infection in the population.

SUBCUTANEOUS: Beneath the skin.

TRANSMISSION: The means by which an infection is transported, or spread, from person to person.

VIRULENCE: The intensity or severity of a disease.

References

1

1. Williams, Stretton, and Leonard (1960).
2. Altman (1990).
3. Altman (1990).
4. Witte, Witte, Minnich, et al. (1984).
5. Altman (1990).
6. Garry, Witte, Gottlieb, et al. (1988).
7. Altman (1990).
8. Katner and Pankey (1987).
9. Rodriguez, Dewhurst, Sinangil, et al. (1985).
10. Panos Institute (1989), p. 35.
11. Grmek (1990) p. 161.
12. Centers for Disease Control (1981a).
13. Centers for Disease Control (1981b).
14. Gottlieb (1991).
15. Centers for Disease Control (1991a).
16. Centers for Disease Control (1990a).
17. Centers for Disease Control (1991a).
18. Centers for Disease Control (1990a).
19. World Health Organization/Centers for Disease Control (1991).

References

20. World Health Organization (1991).
21. Centers for Disease Control (1991b).

2

1. Berkelman and Curran (1989).
2. Fultz (1986).
3. O'Shea et al. (1990).
4. Chiasson et al. (1990).
5. Stewart et al. (1985).
6. Berkelman and Curran (1989).
7. Goedert et al. (1991).
8. European Collaborative Study (1991).
9. Fazakerly and Webb (1985).
10. Berkelman and Curran (1989).
11. Berkelman and Curran (1989).
12. Grmek (1990), p. 89.
13. Panos Institute (1989), p. 27.
14. Berkelman and Curran (1989).
15. Centers for Disease Control (1990b).
16. Berkelman and Curran (1989).
17. Quinn et al. (1988).
18. Eales et al. (1987).
19. Goedert et al. (1991).
20. Koop (1986).

3

1. Centers for Disease Control (1987).
2. Archibald et al. (1986).
3. Major et al. (1991).

5

1. Krasinski and Borkowsky (1991).

6

1. Edinger (1972), pp. 91–96.
2. Kushner (1981), p. 64.

Bibliography

Altman, L. K. (July 24, 1990). Puzzle of sailor's death solved after 31 years: The answer is AIDS. *The New York Times:* C3.

Archibald, D. W., Zon, L. I., Groopman, J. E. et al. (1986). Salivary antibodies as a means of detecting human T cell lymphotropic virus type III/lymphadenopathy-associated virus infection. *Journal of Clinical Microbiology*, 24:873–75.

Berkelman, R. L. and Curran, J. W. (1989). Epidemiology of HIV infection and AIDS. *Epidemiologic Reviews*, 11:222–28.

Centers for Disease Control (1981a). Pneumocystis pneumonia—Los Angeles. *Morbidity and Mortality Weekly Report*, 30: 250–52.

Centers for Disease Control (1981b). Kaposi's sarcoma and pneumocystis pneumonia among homosexual men—New York City and California. *Morbidity and Mortality Weekly Report*, 30: 305–308.

134

Bibliography

Centers for Disease Control (1987). Public health service guidelines for counseling and antibody testing to prevent HIV infection and AIDS. *Morbidity and Mortality Weekly Report,* 36:509–515.

Centers for Disease Control (1990a). HIV prevalence, projected AIDS case estimates: Workshop, October 31–November 1, 1989. *Morbidity and Mortality Weekly Report,* 39:RR-1.

Centers for Disease Control (1990b). Public health service statement on management of occupational exposure to human immunodeficiency virus, including considerations regarding zidovudine postexposure use. *Morbidity and Mortality Weekly Report,* 39:1–14.

Centers for Disease Control (1991a). Mortality attributable to HIV infection/AIDS—United States, 1981–1990. *Morbidity and Mortality Weekly Report,* 40:41–44.

Centers for Disease Control (1991b). The HIV/AIDS epidemic: The first 10 years. *Morbidity and Mortality Weekly Report,* 40:357.

Chiasson, M.A., Stoneburner, R. L., and Joseph, S. C. (1990). Human immunodeficiency virus transmission through artificial insemination. *Journal of Acquired Immune Deficiency Syndromes,* 3:69–72.

Eales, L-J., Nye, K., Parkin, J., et al. (1987). Association of different allelic forms of group specific component with susceptibility to and clinical manifestation of human immunodeficiency virus infection. *Lancet* 2: 999–1002.

Edinger, E. (1972). *Ego and Archetype: Individuation and the Religious Function of the Psyche.* New York: Penguin Books.

European Collaborative Study (1991). Children born to women with HIV-1 infection: Natural history and risk of transmission. *Lancet* 1:253–60.

Bibliography

Fazakerly, J. and Webb, H. (1985). Isolation of AIDS virus from cell-free breast milk of three healthy virus carriers. *Lancet* 2:891–92.

Fultz, P. N. (1986). Components of saliva inactivate human immunodeficiency virus. *Lancet* 2:121.

Garry, R. F., Witte, M. H., Gottlieb, A., et al. (1988). Documentation of an AIDS virus infection in the United States in 1968. *Journal of the American Medical Association,* 260:2085–87.

Goedert, J. J., Duliege, A-M., Amos, C. I., et al. (1991). High risk of HIV-1 infection for first-born twins. *Lancet,* 2:1471–75.

Gottlieb, M. S. (June 5, 1991). Leadership is lacking. *The New York Times:*A15.

Grmek, M. D. (1990). *History of AIDS: Emergence and Origin of a Modern Pandemic.* Princeton, New Jersey: Princeton University Press.

Katner, H. P. and Pankey, G. A. (1987). Evidence for a Euro-American origin of human immunodeficiency virus (HIV). *Journal of the National Medical Association,* 79:1068–72.

Kushner, H. S. (1981). *When Bad Things Happen to Good People.* New York: Schocker Books.

Koop, E. (1986). *Surgeon General's Report on Acquired Immune Deficiency Syndrome.* U.S. Department of Health and Human Services.

Krasinski, K. and Borkowsky, W. (1991). Laboratory diagnosis of HIV infection. *Pediatric Clinics of North America,* 38:17–35.

Major, C., Read, S., Coates, R. et al. (1991). Comparison of saliva and blood for human immunodeficiency virus prevalence testing. *Journal of Infectious Diseases* 163:699–702.

Bibliography

O'Shea, S., Cordery, M., Barrett, W., et al. (1990). HIV excretion patterns and specific antibody responses in body fluids. *Journal of Medical Virology*, 31:291–96.

Panos Institute (1989). *AIDS and the Third World*. Philadelphia: New Society Publishers.

Quinn, T., et al. (1988). Human immunodeficiency virus infection among patients attending clinics for sexually transmitted diseases. *New England Journal of Medicine*, 318:197–203.

Rodriguez, L., Dewhurst, S., Sinangil, F., et al. (1985). Antibodies to HTLV-III/LAV among aboriginal Amazonian Indians in Venezuela. *Lancet*, 2:1098–1100.

Stewart, G. J., Tyler, J. P., Cunningham, A. L., et al. (1985). Transmission of human T-cell lymphotropic virus type III (HTLV-III) by artificial insemination by donor. *Lancet* 2:581–85.

Williams, G., Stretton, T. B., and Leonard, J. C. (1960). Cytomegalic inclusion disease and Pneumocystis carinii infection in an adult. *Lancet* 2:951–55.

Witte, M. H., Witte, C. L., Minnich, L. L., et al. (1984). AIDS in 1968. *Journal of the American Medical Association*, 251:2657.

World Health Organization/Centers for Disease Control (1991). Statistics from the World Health Organization and the Centers for Disease Control. *AIDS*, 5:1043–47.

World Health Organization (1991). *In Point of Fact*. Geneva: World Health Organization (no. 74).

Index

Index

Children
 with AIDS, 13, 15, 16, 28–29
 with HIV infection, 90, 115
 parents lost to AIDS, 16
Community AIDS/HIV testing and
  counseling centers
 counseling, 53, 111, 118, 123
 testing, 44–46, 49, 56, 57, 121,
  123
Confidential testing, 55–56, 60, 64,
  123, 124
Coping
 by loved one with HIV infection,
  102, 103
 when loved one tests positive,
  106–07
 with positive test results, 2, 75–
  99, 118, 120
Coping mechanisms, 77, 78
Costs of testing, 44, 47, 121–22
Counseling, 47, 48, 49–50, 53, 62,
  63, 72, 81, 94
 for depression, 83
 when loved one tests positive,
  106, 107
 testing-site, 45–46, 123, 124
 Counselors, 64, 74, 94–95, 111,
  117, 118, 120

Deaths from AIDS, 13, 15
Denial, 76–77
Depression, 79, 80–84, 87, 110
Discrimination, 12–13, 15, 48, 57,
  64, 122
Drug treatment, 14, 54, 118
Drug use, 87, 89, 92
 see also Intravenous drug use
Drugs, preventive, 51

EIA (Enzyme Immunoassay), 40,
  116
ELISA (Enzyme-Linked Immuno-
  Sorbent Assay), 40–41, 42–43,
  116
Emotional issues, 3, 51, 52 53, 60
  63, 64

awaiting test results, 101–03
negative test results, 68–73
positive test results, 75, 76–87
positive test results in loved one,
  100–01, 103–05
Epidemiology, 42, 59
Europe, 16, 114, 120, 122
European Collaborative Study, 29

False negatives, 67–68, 118
False positives, 43, 117
Family, 79, 97
Fear, 78–84, 107, 110
Federal government, 13, 55, 85
Friends, 79, 97, 100, 101, 112
Frustration, 85–87, 110

Gay-Related Immune Deficiency
  (GRID), 12
Genetic predisposition, 35
Gottlieb, Michael, 11
Guilt, 93–94, 110

Health, 2, 86, 97–98, 111
Health care setting
 risks in, 32–33
Health department clinics, 48–49
Hemophiliacs, 12, 120
Heterosexual sexual acts, 19, 23–25
Heterosexuals, 12, 13, 115
Hispanics, 12, 33, 59–60
HIV (Human Immunodeficiency
  Virus), 1–2, 10–11, 18, 87
 antibody, 38, 73, 119
 contact with, 17, 19, 41, 64,
  120
 defined, 114
 discovery of, 14
 how contracted, 114–15
  (see also Transmission)
 ways not transmitted, 35–36
HIV-1, 14, 114, 120–21
HIV-2, 16, 114, 120–21
HIV-infected persons, 14–15
 social cruelty to, 89–91
 see also Discrimination

140

Index

Index

National Cancer Institute, 28
Needlestick injuries, 32
Negative test results, 40, 41–42, 43, 61, 66, 116
  emotional reactions to, 68–73
  in loved one, 103
  meaning of, 67–68, 118–19
Nonoxynol-9, 21, 24
Nonsexual relations, 101–06
North America
  AIDS epidemic, 10, 11, 12, 114, 115, 120, 122

Opportunistic infections, 14, 39
Oral sex, 21–23, 24, 70
Organ transplants, 19, 30–32
O'Shea, Siobhan, 26

Perinatal transmission, 27–30
Platt, Robert, 8
Pneumocystis pneumonia, 11, 82
Polymerase Chain Reaction (PCR), 43–44, 50, 68
Positive test results, 40–41, 46, 51, 116, 119
  coping with, 2, 75–99, 118, 120
  emotional aftermath of, 3
  emotional preparation for, 64
  fear of facing, 62
  in loved one, 100–13
  meaning of, 117
  penalties for, 55
  privacy concerns, 57
  and retesting, 124
  revealing to others, 122
Pregnancy, 13, 18, 19, 27, 28–30, 33, 111, 115
  planning, 14, 54, 120
Preseminal fluid, 21, 24
Prevention, 18, 45
Privacy issue, 45, 47, 55–56, 57, 64, 105, 122–23
Private physician(s), 46–48, 56, 57, 121, 123
Professional help/support, 63, 64, 94
  see also Counseling; Counselors

Psychological factors, 2–3, 45, 51, 52, 60–63, 76, 102
Psychotherapy, 83
Public education, 13, 25, 45, 116
Public health clinics, 123
Public health department, 55, 58
Public health programs, 1, 33, 59
Punishment, 90, 91–92, 93, 95, 98

Radioimmunoassay, 42
Reagan, Ronald, 13
Reality, 88, 104
  denial of, 76–77
Reconciliation, 76, 87, 89, 93, 95–96
Relationships
  when both test positive, 107–11
  intimate, 54, 59
  and positive test results, 97, 100–13
  terminating, 106–07, 108
  see also Lovers; Spouse
Relatives, 97, 100, 101, 112
Renewal, 96–99
Reporting practices, 57–59, 127–28
Resources, 125–26
Responsibility, 16–17, 71, 86
Retesting, 41, 50, 73, 74, 77, 119, 124
Rimming, 26
Risk factors, 18–36, 53, 116
Risky behavior, 12, 71

Sadomasochism, 26
Saliva, 20, 22, 25–26
Saliva tests, 42–43
Self-image/respect, 79, 86–87, 93
Semen, 20, 21, 24, 25, 26, 27, 34, 114–15
Sex, 10, 87
  safe, 25, 110
  unsafe, 12, 34, 120
Sex industry, 58–59, 120
Sexual activity
  transmission through, 18, 19, 20–27, 89, 91, 93, 115

Index

About the Author

MARC VARGO earned a Master of Science degree in clinical psychology from Murray State University, pursued advanced studies at the California School of Professional Psychology, and completed the predoctoral internship in clinical psychology at the School of Medicine, Louisiana State University. His research, which has focused primarily on death anxiety, has been published in several American and European professional journals.

Since 1987 Mr. Vargo has been associated with the NO/AIDS Task Force (New Orleans), providing gratis services as an HIV counselor and, at one point, serving as chairperson of its HIV counseling program. He has also been associated with the New Orleans AIDS Project, a federally funded community service program, through which he facilitated support groups for infected individuals.

At present, Mr. Vargo is employed by Hammond Developmental Center. He resides in the French Quarter of New Orleans and continues to provide HIV-related psychological services in the metropolitan area.